The Core Workout

A Definitive Guide to Swiss Ball Training for Athletes, Coaches & Fitness Professionals

Fourth Edition

Joanne Elphinston & Paul Pook

Lincoln College

2001027

Copyright © 2010 by Joanne Elphinston and Paul Pook. All rights reserved. No portion of this book, except for brief review, may be reproduced, stored in a retrieval system, or transmitted in any form or by any means – electronic, mechanical, photocopying, recording, or otherwise – without the written permission of the publisher. For information, contact Lotus Publishing.

First published in 1998 by Core Workout. Second edition published in 2000, and third edition published in 2004.
This fourth edition published in 2010 by
Lotus Publishing, Apple Tree Cottage, Inlands Road, Nutbourne, Chichester, PO18 8RJ, UK.

Disclaimer

The training programme in this manual has been devised with safety as its priority. The authors advocate careful, responsible use of the ball. The Safety Check and Medical History section is provided as a guide but in no way replaces the supervision of a trained medical professional. The authors and publisher cannot be held liable for injuries sustained during *The Core Workout*, or by misuse or misunderstanding associated with the material herein.

Illustrations Amanda Williams
Photographs Scanpix, istock
Cover Design Richard Evans
Text Design Wendy Craig
Printed and Bound in the UK by Scotprint

British Library Cataloguing in Publication Data
A CIP record for this book is available from the British Library
ISBN 978 1 905367 10 8

ENTRE	Newark
CHECKED	CR
ZONE	Purple
SHELF MARK / PREFIX	613.7 ELP
LOAN PERIOD	1 Week

2001027
716.c1

Contents

Preface

The concept of core stability has become a fundamental element in sports training practice, as athletes seek methods to reduce stress on their bodies and optimise their physical performance. However, sometimes it is difficult to find effective and motivating methods to integrate core stability training into existing programmes. It was with this in mind that we produced *The Core Workout*, which is based on our experiences in training a wide variety of elite athletes and sportspeople in core stability and movement efficiency.

Initially, we began to work together with the purpose of combining our different professional backgrounds of physiotherapy and sport science, aiming to develop safe and effective training strategies for performance enhancement. An integral part of this approach has been Swiss Ball training, as we have found over time that we can tailor a core stability programme from the very basic to the very advanced, that athlete compliance is excellent because the ball is challenging and fun to work with, and that it allows us many alternatives if an athlete is injured. We have also found the ball to be particularly useful in team training and group situations, which has led to the original exercises presented in the Double Trouble section of this manual.

The Core Workout was originally a record of our ideas and development as our applications to different sporting needs expanded, but over time the demand from various sporting bodies and individual sportspeople increased for a text from which they can work and progress. Despite originally pitching the book at the higher level sports training market, it has been unexpected and pleasing to find that Levels 1 and 2 in the 'Library of Exercises' of the original book have been used effectively by its readers to sort out their aches and pains as well, so thank you to those who have emailed us over the years to tell us about your successes. The ball's versatility in a rehabilitation setting is limitless; however it is not within the scope of this manual to adequately and specifically address this topic, despite the strong temptation to do so!

As a final note, the Swiss Ball is a versatile tool for training and is currently being used at very high levels for training in a wide range of sports. We have international sprinters, rugby players, archers, surfers, golfers and martial artists training on balls to name but a few, and combined with a better understanding of their own body movement and function, they are experiencing excellent results. We encourage you to use the ball with a bit of imagination and creativity, and hope that equipped with the principles which are introduced here, you will find ways to make it a relevant and valuable part of your training.

Core Stability for Sport and Conditioning

Strength, speed, flexibility and agility are among the fitness parameters commonly trained to make you effective in sport. The type of sport or the position in which you play will affect the relative balance of these qualities, but whether it is in a team sport or downhill skiing, you are ultimately aiming for a combination which will lead to physical control and optimal performance.

Training often focuses on obvious, easily visible muscle groups in the arms and legs. While the relationship between these muscles and the movements of the limbs is readily accepted, e.g. hamstring muscles and the knee bending movement, what is overlooked is an understanding that these muscles of the limbs depend on a solid foundation to pull from for their effectiveness. Training core stability develops this foundation.

What is Core Stability?

Core stability provides central body control, and allows you to generate power by maximising the efficiency of your muscular effort. **It is the ability of your trunk to support and withstand the forces acting upon it, including those created by your arms and legs, in order that the muscles and joints can perform in their safest, strongest and most effective positions.**

Your core is not just your back, but also the pelvic and shoulder girdles, which are responsible for transferring forces between your limbs and your trunk. The shoulder girdle is made up of your collarbones and your shoulder-blades, and provides an anchor for your arm movements via muscular attachments to your midback and rib cage. The pelvic girdle functions in a similar manner, with the abdominal and gluteal muscles working to maintain its position relative to the spine. This allows the pelvis to provide a stable base for your legs to pull from.

If the wrong muscles are activated to transfer the forces from your limbs through these girdles to your spine, or if the appropriate muscles work but are relatively weak, the body will try to find a way to compensate. It does this by adjusting other parts of the body into positions that are not necessarily ideal for the demands of the movement. When this occurs, you lose efficiency, and this translates into a loss of power. It can also make you vulnerable to injuries such as shoulder tendonitis or lower back pain.

The muscles responsible for optimal force transfer between the limbs and the trunk, i.e. those that stabilise your central body, or **core**, are therefore essential for optimal body functioning. This force transfer is a necessary part of movement, and you can improve the way in which it happens to make it safe and efficient. It doesn't matter how much weight training you do on your arms and legs: **you can only be as strong as your weakest link, and if that link is your core stability, it needs to be integrated into your training.**

How Can Core Stability Improve My Performance?

By training for core stability, you can gain a number of benefits:
- More efficient use of muscle power, as less effort is lost in compensatory movements
- Decreased injury risk, as forces are managed by the appropriate body structures
- Improved ability to change direction, as body momentum is more effectively controlled
- Greater capacity for speed generation as power muscles have a secure platform to pull from
- Improved balance and muscular coordination
- Improved posture

How Do I Train for Core Stability?

You need to train specifically for the tasks required. In other words, you train the stabilising muscles to hold the trunk and girdles steady while you introduce resistance from the arms, legs, or gravity. For example, the abdominal muscles, key stabilisers, are often only trained with sit-ups, and this trunk curling movement does not necessarily relate to the abdominals' role in supporting your trunk while running, swinging a golf club, or changing direction quickly. By performing sit-ups you would be training the abdominals as **mobilisers**, muscles which create motion, as opposed to training the muscles as **stabilisers**, those which support and hold against the forces of the moving limbs.

Bodies also need to be trained to work effectively in multiple planes of movement. Many common exercises focus on one plane at a time, for example bench-pressing on a machine, but in reality the body is often required to work in multiple planes. The body in sport constantly moves through combinations of joint rotation, often incorporating the trunk and limbs simultaneously. This rotation is necessary for full functional range of motion, and also for 'winding up' the muscles so that they temporarily store energy for movement, something like twisting up a rubber band and then seeing the quick movement it produces when released.

The core stabilising muscles are responsible for controlling these rotatory forces; however this control does not develop by repeatedly performing movements in one plane, especially when fully supported. Exercising on an unstable base like the exercise ball helps to stimulate multidirectional control, and helps to 'wake up' the core stabilisers.

Core Stability and Lower Back Pain

Recent research has shown that the muscles responsible for supporting the lower back are the very muscles that stop working effectively in the presence of pain. Whether you are involved in an athletic pursuit or not, these muscles are necessary to control movement of the trunk and limbs, and limit excessive stress on the spine.

The principles outlined for sports performance therefore also apply in the case of back pain. Development of a coordinated, stable trunk or 'core' is essential to recover from a back injury, even if you just want to return to everyday tasks. Control of movement in many planes is part of normal activity, and training the body to activate the stabilising muscles and then to respond to an unstable surface such as the ball can contribute to this process.

At first, activating the stabilisers can take a bit of 'brain work' – you have to develop a relationship with muscles that you may not be familiar with. This isn't always easy! Developing core stability will initially require mental focus to become aware of your body position and posture, but gradually over time this and the corresponding muscle actions will become more automatic.

The Core Muscles

Abdominals

It comes as a surprise to most people that the abdominals are not just one muscle, but are in fact made up of the rectus abdominis, internal and external obliques, and transversus abdominis muscles. These muscles all have a different action and function. Athletes spend a great deal of time training one or two muscles, often with standard sit-ups and perhaps sit-ups with a twist, but never access the critically important abdominal muscle which gives the deepest support for the spine – the transversus abdominis, or trans abs. This muscle wraps around the entire trunk wall and inserts at the back into a strong, broad structure called the thoraco-lumbar fascia. It plays a primary role in keeping the lumbar spine and pelvis stable during movement.

ABDOMINAL MUSCLES

TRANS ABS INSERTING INTO THE THORACO-LUMBAR FASCIA

Gluteals

The muscles around your hip and bottom are not just for sitting on – these muscles are extremely important power *generators*. The gluteus maximus (or 'glute max') is activated whenever the hip must move between bending and straightening. This means it has a key role in **speed** (think of the prominent buttocks which you see on top sprinters), **lifting** whether it is in a lineout or a dead lift, jumping forwards or upwards, **controlling** a landing, or even contributing to **balance** as a lawn bowler steps forwards!

If you are involved in a propulsive sport such as basketball, football or sprinting, think of glute max as an 'engine' which drives your body forwards and upwards. If your sport requires accuracy and defined movements, the gluteal group of muscles increases control and contributes to a stable base from which to shoot, swing, kick or balance. Many of our clients, regardless of their sport, lack appropriate activation in their glutes to adequately control their hip, knee or back, and not only risk injury, but are unable to perform to their potential.

Gluteus maximus

Necessary for powerful extension of the hip

Other muscles of this region, such as gluteus medius, are responsible for side to side stability of the pelvis as well as sideways leg movement. Without this muscle functioning properly, you cannot stand on one leg without your pelvis tipping, leading to compensatory side bending of your spine and excess stress to the lower back or other parts of the pelvis, once again decreasing efficiency and risking injury.

Inadequate Stability

If Gluteus medius is weak, the pelvis may tip when weight bearing on that side

Adequate Stability

With better hip abductor function, the pelvis remains level on weight bearing

HIP ABDUCTOR FUNCTION

The gluteals are also critical in the support of the lower back, and are often found to be weak, under-active or uncoordinated in individuals with lower back pain. If this is the case, you may tend to overuse your back and knees to make up for the weakness, and even everyday activities such as climbing stairs and getting out of a chair can be affected.

There are numerous smaller muscles in the hip region that have important roles to play in stability, and throughout *The Core Workout* they will be activated to assist the larger muscles to control your hip and knee position. The gluteals, however, need particular attention, as problems with these muscles can contribute to back, knee and groin injuries.

Upper Body Stability

In the upper body, the core muscles are just as important. Just as the abdominals and gluteals contribute to and help control lower limb and back movement, another set of muscles performs the same role for the upper limb. In order for you to be able to move your arm, the muscles responsible for the movement must have a stable base to pull from. This base is your shoulder-blade, or scapula. However, to fulfil this role, the scapula must be fixed to the trunk in some way, otherwise the force will be lost from your arm movement.

The muscles that are responsible for this scapular control are the upper and lower trapezius, which attach to the skull and larger bones of the lower midback, and the serratus anterior, which attaches to the ribs. These attachments give a relatively large surface area to support arm forces, and combine to angulate the scapula upwards, giving the 'ball' of the ball-and-socket joint of the shoulder room to rotate in the movement of lifting the arm.

POOR STABILISING PATTERN
FORCES SENT TO NECK AND UPPER BACK
(SMALL SURFACE AREA)

IDEAL STABILISING PATTERN
FORCES SHED ACROSS
BROAD SURFACE AREA

Often, however, we see athletes who do not use this pattern to achieve arm movement. Instead of staying flat on the rib cage, their scapulae lift off or 'wing', and neck and upper back muscles pull the scapula upwards. This has two effects. The first is that arm power decreases, as the forces are sent to smaller, weaker areas such as the neck. The second is that injury risk is increased, both in the joints of the neck, as well as the tendons of the shoulder. If the scapula does not angulate upwards, there is a risk that the tendons of your shoulder will be compressed, leading to painful tendonitis.

Once the scapula is well positioned to provide a good 'socket' angle, the muscles of the rotator cuff help to control the movement of the 'ball' of the shoulder joint. These muscles have a critical role to play, ensuring that the rolling and sliding motion of normal shoulder movement does not deviate forwards or upwards within the socket. Core Workout exercises involving the arms demand a great deal of stabilising muscle activity around the shoulder and if you maintain good body position, Swiss Ball training can stimulate and strengthen the rotator cuff.

It is not just the rotator cuff and scapular muscles that protect and support the shoulder. The pelvic muscles and trunk stabilisers are absolutely critical, as it is these that provide the foundation necessary for a good shoulder position. When working on your shoulders, always pay attention to controlling your pelvic and trunk position, as this will best place your shoulder in order to activate a coordinated muscle pattern.

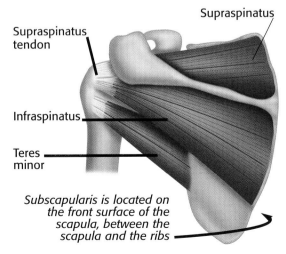

BACK VIEW OF THE LEFT SHOULDER
ROTATOR CUFF MUSCLES

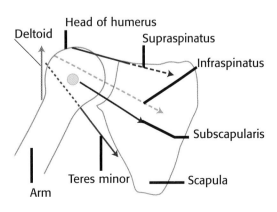

ROTATOR CUFF ACTION SECURES THE
'BALL' IN THE 'SOCKET'

Summary

Training for athletic performance has become considerably more sophisticated in recent years. For both athletes and sports professionals, the time has passed when 'doing what we've always done' is acceptable, just as using exercises and techniques without understanding how or why they are supposed to work is not good practice. Increasingly, a knowledge of how the body functions, along with a good grasp of the specific physical and psychological demands of the sport is necessary to really achieve results and avoid injury over time.

There are several principles that shape a programme for core stability:

Understand the demands of your sport

Training may focus on a selection of characteristics, but perhaps not consider the interplay between them. Ask yourself what the sport breaks down into for the individual player or athlete, e.g. linear speed, rapid change of direction, upwards or forwards explosive power, rotational control, blocking the forces of other players, ability to stop suddenly, ability to balance in a variety of body positions, ability to control ballistic actions of the upper and lower limbs, etc. If the sport requires a complex movement, such as in gymnastics or power lifting, make sure that you have a clear understanding of how such a movement is achieved.

Develop an understanding of basic anatomy and muscle actions

If you understand how your body works, it will subtly alter how you perform your movements, and help to focus your mind on what you are doing. For example, an athlete with a poor concept of muscle action and inadequate training objectives may decide to perform a bicep curl to increase bicep strength, but fails to focus on which muscles are responsible for movement, and which muscles are necessary for support. He or she simply aims to 'get the weight up', which leads to the use of momentum (swinging) combined with back motion to lift the weight. The whole body starts to move, instead of what should be a simple elbow bending movement using concentrated biceps brachii muscle effort founded on a stabilised shoulder-blade and trunk for correct support. The result of this lack of understanding is a relatively poor outcome for the effort and time spent, and a further safety risk.

Train muscles specifically for their role in your sport

If the muscle should stabilise, train it for that role whenever you train the mobilising muscles which it should support. Also remember that in sport, balance and quick muscle reactions in multiple planes are required, and that these features should be built upon a foundation of core stability.

The Swiss Ball

Although the Swiss Ball has been around since the 1930s, its potential for training rather than just rehabilitation had not been explored until relatively recently. The major advantage of Swiss Ball training is that it provides an unstable support surface, which stimulates the body's stabilising mechanisms. This allows you to train the function of the muscles and not just their strength. The Swiss Ball is extremely versatile, and can be used for a variety of purposes. It allows for integrated 'whole body' exercise, from low levels through to high levels, and combines well with other forms of training.

Equipment Guidelines

Do not inflate your ball over the maximum prescribed diameter. The correct diameter is the same as the size indicated on the ball. This is the **maximum** diameter of the ball.

To Inflate

Manufacturers recommend that the ball should be half inflated overnight, and then topped up the next day so that the fabric of the ball is allowed to expand gently.

1. Mark the indicated height of the ball on a wall so that you have an idea what you are aiming for. This will be a guideline for the suggested size of the inflated ball, but not an absolute measure.
2. Remove the plug from the ball and inflate with a manual pump or air compressor. Do not over inflate, otherwise the fabric of the ball may become damaged. The ball should feel firm but not hard.
3. Measure the ball against the marked indicator on the wall. You may find that the ball is firm but is not the same size as the marked height. Some are a little smaller, and some a little larger depending upon the make and fabric. Make your judgement based on feel. There should not be too much 'give' in the ball, and nor should it feel completely solid.
4. To deflate your Swiss Ball, remove the plug carefully by exerting a pulling pressure while moving the plug back and forth.

Basic Safety

1. Use only on a safe level ground, preferably on a non-slip surface such as a yoga mat
2. Wear shoes with non-slip soles
3. Avoid contact with sharp objects or sources of heat such as central heating radiators
4. Make sure that your practice space is clear and unobstructed
5. Do not use near stairs
6. Small parts such as the plugs may be easily swallowed, so care should be taken with small children

Basic Guidelines

To perform *The Core Workout* safely and for optimal results, there are several basic principles that must be understood.

Neutral Alignment

Neutral alignment allows the joints and muscles to perform at their best with the least risk of injury. This neutral alignment must be maintained throughout the movements in *The Core Workout*. Your key areas of focus are the neck, shoulder-blades, pelvis, knees and feet. Deviations from neutral not only decrease your body's efficiency, but also increase your potential for injury and body pain.

To find your neutral position, stand relaxed, and then draw yourself up from the back of your head, lengthening and relaxing your spine. Your posture should change automatically in a number of ways. Notice that your chin may lower slightly and the back of your neck may flatten slightly. Your shoulders should be relaxed down away from your ears, and not too far forwards. Your pelvis should be level under your shoulders, and your stomach will have drawn in slightly.

Lengthen through the back of your neck

Relaxed shoulders

Hips under shoulders

POOR POSTURE   IMPROVED POSTURE

These positions should be maintained whether you are standing, sitting, on your back...

LYING SUPINE ON THE BALL

...or on your front.

LYING PRONE ON THE BALL

Stomach Scooping

A key concept to master is **stomach scooping**. Drawing the very lower part of your belly back and slightly up as if 'scooping it' towards your spine activates your transversus abdominis muscle, otherwise known as the 'trans abs.' This muscle contributes to the stability of your trunk, helping to create a foundation for more powerful arm and leg movements.

To finds your trans abs, place your hand on your lower belly and draw yourself up from the back of your head as outlined in 'neutral alignment.' You will find that this action will automatically bring the stomach in, allowing the body to lengthen and narrow through the waist area. Now slowly raise an arm above your head, keeping the feeling of being long, straight and narrow through the waist, and you should find that the stomach draws in a little more in order to prevent your spine from sagging forwards. Maintain that sensation while lowering your arm. Your transversus abdominis allows your limbs to move while keeping the spine in a safe, efficient position.

The concept of lengthening and narrowing is very important to sustain, particularly as the exercises become more challenging. It is tempting to use other muscles which give an impression of abdominal tautness, but which pull the rib cage down towards the pubic bone. If you feel as if you are 'compressing' or 'gripping' your middle, you are not using your trans abs.

Getting in touch with your trans abs may be difficult, and different ways of accessing them may be necessary at first. Here are several other methods for further developing your awareness of trans abs.

Begin by lying on your back with your knees bent. Breathe out fully, and before breathing in, draw the lower stomach back towards the spine, as if scooping the area below the belly button back and slightly upwards. Sustain this contraction, and proceed with breathing.

If you have difficulty breathing, place your hands on your lower ribs, and make sure that as you breathe in, your ribs expand under your hands, and as you breathe out, that your ribs ease back in again. You should be able to do this while maintaining the 'scooping' feeling in your lower abdominals.

Lie on your back or side. Imagine pulling your tailbone towards your pubic bone, activating the muscles between them, and then pull those muscles upwards as if into the very lower abdominals just above the pubic bone. Sustain this contraction and continue to breathe.

 Take up a position with your hands on knees, so that your hands are directly under your shoulders and your knees are under your hips. Focus on the very lower part of your belly, and scoop it upwards towards your spine. Continue to breathe while sustaining the contraction.

This is a very small muscle contraction, so when activating trans abs, the rest of your body should be relaxed, i.e. your shoulders and ribs should not feel awkward, and your back muscles should not be tense.

Stomach scooping is an essential part of all core movements.

ATHLETE WITH POOR POSTURE AND SAGGING STOMACH

ATHLETE IN 'DRAWN UP' POSTURE WITH BETTER ALIGNMENT AND TRANS ABS ACTIVITY

The movement comes from the stomach, not the ribs or shoulders. Becoming more active in the abdominals should not cause you to raise your shoulders or your rib cage.

Power Zones

It is helpful to think of your body as having **three power zones**. When using your arms, the forces need to be directed into the **upper** power zone. This is an imaginary circle at mid-chest level, and includes the stabilising muscles that transmit the arm forces to the midback, as well as the rotator cuff.

If you allow your arm forces to be directed *above* your upper power zone, they will be transmitted through longer, thinner muscles to the neck, decreasing the power potential of the arms and increasing the risk of neck pain.

UPPER POWER ZONE

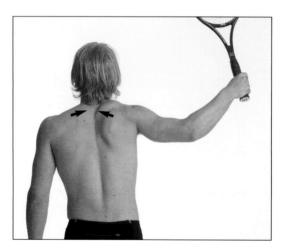

PLAYER ATTEMPTING TO STABILISE HIS SHOULDER-BLADE (SCAPULA) BY ELEVATING IT. FORCES ARE THEN DIRECTED TO THE NECK

IMPROVED SHOULDER-BLADE POSITION. FORCES DIRECTED INTO MIDBACK

The **central** power zone is a 'corset' that loops around the area between your ribs and your pelvis. When moving your legs (and arms in some circumstances), this corset acts to stop the forces from being converted into harmful, excessive spinal movements. Visualise a strong cylinder around this area and maintain it throughout each exercise.

CENTRAL POWER ZONE

LOWER POWER ZONE

The **lower** power zone controls the pelvis and thigh, and utilizes the gluteal group of muscles. The lower power zone enables you to keep your pelvis level and your spine aligned, which can help to decrease the risk of knee and pelvic injury. Visualise a firm ring encircling the pelvis: when using your lower body, imagine keeping this ring level, and containing your forces between the ring and your feet.

When performing *The Core Workout*, try to focus on these power zones. If you feel excessive tension in your neck or lower back, relax these areas and concentrate on the muscles in the 'power zones', to provide the support necessary for the exercise that you are performing.

Mental Cues

Above all, it is important to use the correct mental cues for this type of work. The words that go through your mind as you think about an exercise can influence how you perform it, and can change the programming from your brain to your body.

As we have already discussed, words like 'gripping' or 'clenching' the muscles are likely to activate unwanted muscles. Instead, words like 'lengthening', 'narrowing' and 'releasing' are more helpful. The most important cue however, is 'effortless' control. If you see a world-class sprinter in action you will notice the relaxation around their shoulders and neck, even though they are performing to their maximum ability. A less talented athlete will appear to be using a great deal of effort, which will be evident in excessive tension throughout their body.

Greater effort during a movement does not necessarily facilitate a great performance. Visualise yourself performing with the same level of effortlessness that you see in elite athletes by keeping in mind the cue of 'effortless' control.

Breathing

It is common to hold your breath when learning the core exercises and this is partly to do with concentration and effort. However, it is not a helpful strategy for developing stability, as the breath and breathing muscles are normally closely coordinated with effective transversus abdominis function.

Remind yourself to smoothly continue breathing throughout an exercise, and that you are aiming for effortless control. If you are having difficulty doing this, try using your voice by counting out loud or repeating a phrase as you perform the exercise so that breathing and body control occur together naturally.

Pain

Exercises with the ball should make your muscles feel as though they are working, but should not cause pain. If you experience pain during an exercise, consult your doctor or physiotherapist.

Warm-up and Cool-down

It is advisable that you warm-up prior to starting *The Core Workout*. Several minutes of light aerobic exercise and progressive stretching (see pages 118–127) will prepare your joints and muscles.

When you have finished *The Core Workout*, you are advised to cool-down by repeating the stretches you performed during the warm-up. This will reduce the likelihood of muscle soreness.

Warm-up ▶ Stretch ▶ **The Core Workout** ▶ Cool-down ▶ Stretch

Common Errors

There are several common errors that will decrease the effectiveness of the movements. These are illustrated on pages 23–26.

Back Arching

Notice that the hips are raised too high. This is because the back muscles are being used instead of the bottom (glutes). This usually happens when the glutes are either not strong enough, not activating appropriately, or the athlete has a poor movement pattern which has developed over time.

BACK ARCHING   NEUTRAL SPINAL POSITION

If you are having difficulty achieving a level position without back strain, try bending your hips a little and then tilt your pelvis slightly back towards you until you feel your back relax and your bottom tighten.

Shoulder Hitching

The shoulders need to stay low, 'away from your ears' to keep the forces from your arms directed into your upper 'power zone' at mid-chest level.

 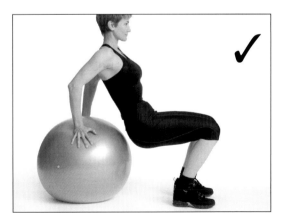

SHOULDER HITCHING   NEUTRAL SHOULDER POSITION

Allowing the shoulders to creep up increases stress on the shoulder joints and sends potential harmful forces to the neck.

Chin Poking

Poking of the chin is another compensatory manoeuvre that reinforces poor postural habits and can affect the biomechanics of the neck, shoulders and trunk.

CHIN POKING

CORRECT CHIN POSITION

Knees Deviating Inwards

This error occurs when the muscles of the side and back of the hips (gluteals) fail to control the angle of the thigh (femur).

Concentrate on the muscles that should be performing the movement.

KNEES DEVIATING INWARDS

CORRECT KNEE ALIGNMENT

Hip Flexing

This tends to occur when the abdominals are unable to hold the trunk in neutral. The relatively strong hip flexors are recruited to prevent the back from sagging, but this error will prevent development of the abdominals as stabilisers.

HIP FLEXING   NEUTRAL HIP ALIGNMENT

Back Sagging

This also occurs when the abdominals do not function adequately to keep the trunk position neutral, but in the case illustrated, the hip trunk flexors are not compensating.

BACK SAGGING

Stomach Protruding

If your transversus abdominis is not active during an exercise, you will notice that the middle part of the abdominal wall will protrude, as demonstrated below. This is your rectus abdominis muscle, and it tends to act excessively if your trans abs are not activating correctly. This leads to a muscle imbalance and loss of core stability.

PREDOMINANT RECTUS ABDOMINIS

IMPROVED PATTERN USING TRANS ABS

Form is Everything

The most important principle is this: form is everything. You will not benefit from performing the movements too hard, fast or far for your capabilities. This type of training targets subtle muscles and coordination, and if you disregard the principle of form, you will not progress. Worse still, it may create a risk of injury.

ATHLETE BEYOND HIS CAPABILITIES

This is an example of an athlete who has gone beyond his capabilities, and has lost neutral alignment. As you can see, the back is sagging, the neck is not in neutral alignment, and the hips are flexed. The athlete is gaining no benefit from this exercise, and risks injury.

Safety Check and Medical History

This workout is designed for healthy athletes and fitness enthusiasts. If you are recovering from an injury, we recommend the guidance of a health professional when beginning a rehabilitation programme, and that you limit your initial exercise choice to exercises which appear in the 'Getting Started' or Level 1 categories. Use of the Swiss Exercise Ball is highly appropriate for all levels of fitness and rehabilitation, but some of the exercises outlined in *The Core Workout* are relatively advanced, and are aimed at high level conditioning only.

It is important that you consider your health status prior to following *The Core Workout* and using the Swiss Exercise Ball. Exercise involves the risk of injury. If you are in any doubt about your current state of health or how vulnerable you are to injury, seek medical advice before following this programme.

You are advised to complete the following Medical History Questionnaire and if any of your responses are positive, please consult your health professional before following *The Core Workout.*

Medical History Questionnaire

1. Have you ever suffered from any form of heart complaint?
2. Is there any history of heart disease in your family?
3. Have you ever suffered from epilepsy?
4. Are you recovering from an illness or operation?
5. Have you ever had asthma or suffered from any breathing difficulties?
6. Are you presently taking any form of medication?
7. Are you diabetic?
8. Do you currently have any form of muscle or joint injury?
9. Is there any other reason why it may be inadvisable for you to perform *The Core Workout*?

Any 'Yes' Answers?
You should consult your doctor before performing the exercises outlined in *The Core Workout.* Check that it is safe for you to go ahead.

Progression of Exercises

There are many methods for progressing Swiss Ball exercises, but the most significant influences are:

1. Base of Support
2. Planes of Movement
3. Length of Lever

Base of Support

The amount of space taken up by the body as it contacts the floor or the wall is the size of the base of support. The base of support can be increased or decreased by widening or narrowing foot or arm contact with the floor or wall. A wider base is more stable and therefore makes an exercise easier. A narrow base provides less stability and is therefore more challenging to control.

FLOOR BRIDGE USING ARMS TO CREATE A WIDER BASE BY INCREASING SURFACE CONTACT

FLOOR BRIDGE WITH ARMS ACROSS CHEST WHICH NARROWS THE BASE BY DECREASING SURFACE CONTACT

WALL-PRESS WITH FEET APART TO CREATE A WIDE BASE

WALL-PRESS WITH FEET TOGETHER TO NARROW THE BASE OF SUPPORT.

WALL-PRESS ON SINGLE LEG TO FURTHER NARROW THE BASE OF SUPPORT

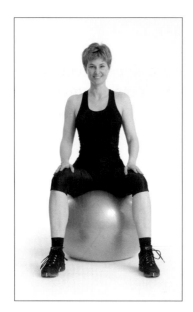

SEATED WITH FEET
APART IS MORE STABLE

SEATED WITH FEET TOGETHER NARROWS THE BASE OF SUPPORT
AND IS THEREFORE MORE CHALLENGING TO CONTROL.

Planes of Movement

The direction in which you move your arms will influence the difficulty of the exercise. In exercises such as Floor Bridge, Suspension Bridge and Superman, these arm movement planes will alter the challenge for the trunk stabilisers, especially when a small hand weight is introduced.

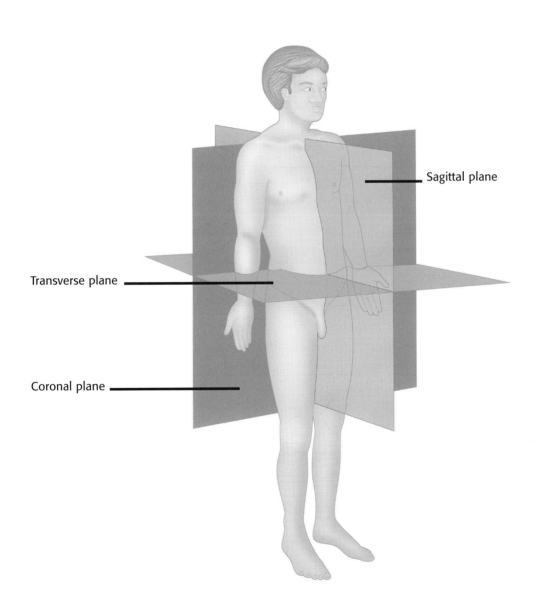

Sagittal plane

Transverse plane

Coronal plane

The Sagittal Plane

The sagittal plane is the forwards and backwards plane. Moving your arms or leg in line with your body is usually the easiest direction to control.

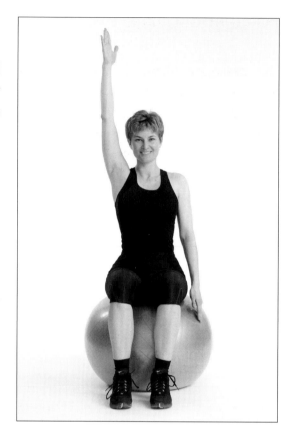

The Coronal Plane

The coronal plane is the side movement plane. Moving your arms in a sideways arc away from your body is easy to control if the movement is done symmetrically (both arms together), but if done with only one arm, this plane is more difficult to control.

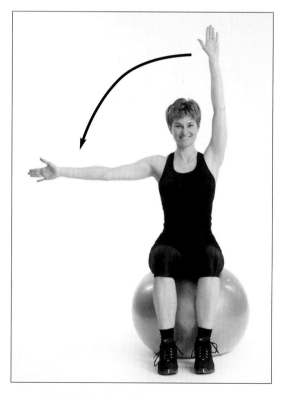

ASYMMETRICAL CORONAL MOVEMENT

The Transverse Plane

The transverse plane is the rotational movement plane. If both arms move symmetrically in an outward arc, the forces on the body are balanced and the movement is easily controlled. However, this is the most challenging plane to control if only one arm is moved.

ASYMMETRICAL TRANSVERSE MOVEMENT IN SEATED POSITION

SYMMETRICAL TRANSVERSE MOVEMENT IN SUSPENSION BRIDGE POSITION

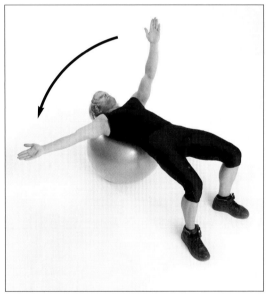

ASYMMETRICAL TRANSVERSE MOVEMENT IN SUSPENSION BRIDGE POSITION

Length of Lever

The length of lever is the distance of the ball from your surface contact point. The balance and stability challenge on the trunk increases as the ball moves further from the surface contact point.

Changing the lever is a powerful way to increase exercise difficulty: you only need to change the lever by a small amount to increase the trunk demand.

LENGTHENING THE LEVER BY MOVING THE BALL FURTHER FROM THE CONTACT POINT

THE SAME PRINCIPLE APPLIES IN THE OVER THE TOP POSITION

In standing, the lever is lengthened by moving further from the wall. The stability demand on the body is increased with even a small lever change.

In Suspension Bridge however, the head must always be correctly supported with the neck in neutral, so lever changes must be done by taking the arms over the head rather than moving the feet away from the ball.

Other Progression Methods

Options such as performing exercises with eyes closed, throwing and catching balls, or combining with other equipment such as balance boards or hand weights can also increase the balance and stability challenge of your Swiss Ball exercise.

Getting Started

This is a collection of exercises which teaches you to pay attention to how your body moves. Some exercises focus on the upper body primarily and others emphasise the lower body. However in all of the exercises, attention to full body alignment is essential to maximise benefit. Exercise ball work should be viewed as 'whole body' exercise.

These are also good movements to practice when beginning rehabilitation after a back injury. Remember to consult your physiotherapist when undertaking exercise after injury.

As with all ball exercises, these movements need to be performed slowly and with good quality. Begin with only four or five repetitions, as you will tire quickly, and this will lead to poor movement. As you become better at the movements, you can start to increase your repetitions. Your target is ten quality repetitions.

A special note: *Athletes often think that these exercises will be too easy, and try to skip over them. Unfortunately, very few of the sportsmen and sportswomen whom we see can perform these exercises well, especially when we slow them down to really see what's going on. No matter how high your athletic ability, it is important that you start to develop an awareness of your body's stabilising systems, and these movements will give you the opportunity to do so.* Remember: Form is everything!

1. Seated Arm Raise

This exercise is performed most effectively in front of a mirror.

START POSITION

RAISED ARM POSITION

POOR STABILITY POSITION

Sit with your knees in line with your feet, and your spine in the neutral position. Slowly raise one arm, and watch whether your trunk bends, or the ball moves. If it does, try lengthening your trunk as you lift, and draw your tummy in to control the movement. You should feel an increased tension in the abdomen as your arm approaches its highest point. Now try alternating arms. There should be no sideways trunk movement, no back arching, and no shoulder hitching.

Now try both arms over your head – your spine should stay in its neutral position.

NEUTRAL POSITION   EXTENSION COMPENSATION   FLEXION COMPENSATION

To increase the difficulty, start with your feet closer together, but not quite touching. This will decrease your base of support and create a greater stability challenge.

2. Single Leg Raise

Sit in the neutral position, with your feet together. Scoop your lower abdomen slightly in and 'under your tummy button', so that it can assist in stabilising your trunk. Now slowly peel one foot off the floor, bending at the hip joint, not at the waist. Replace the foot, and repeat with the other side.

START POSITION

CORRECT FINISH POSITION

3. Combination Lift

If you have mastered 1. and 2., try starting with your arms above your head, and lift one foot from the floor.

Your trunk should stay in its neutral position as you lift the foot. Make sure that you don't shorten one side to make it easier!

CORRECT POSITION
(NEUTRAL SPINE)

POOR POSITION
(FLEXED SPINE)

4. Ab Exploration

This exercise allows you to notice how the abdominal muscles respond to stresses in different directions. Your aim is to keep your back resting comfortably on the floor throughout all movements, and therefore to avoid tipping or arching of the back.

Lie on your back with your knees bent and the ball in your hands. Gently perform a stomach scoop, and push the ball up towards the ceiling. Now slowly move the ball a small distance over your head: at some point you may feel that your back needs to arch, and at that point you need to narrow and lengthen at the waist and 'scoop' your abdominals a little more to control that movement.

Now try moving the ball a little to the left, and then a little to the right. Feel the abdominals respond to keep control of your trunk. Then experiment with diagonals, from over the right shoulder across the body to the left hip, and vice-versa. If you find that you are better in some directions than others, emphasise the directions which need 'topping up'.

Now move the ball in a circle, feeling the muscle response in your abdomen shift in a corresponding circle. To increase the loading, increase the size of the circle.

Ensure that your back is lengthened and relaxed, that you are stomach scooping, and that your trunk is resting symmetrically on the floor throughout all movements. The slower you go, the more you notice and the more effective the exercise is for your abdominals.

5. Neutral Bounce

It is important to learn to control the spine while in motion. Many athletes allow their spines to buckle or arch once a dynamic movement is introduced. The seated bounce trains you to recognise and consistently control a neutral spinal position.

Find a neutral spinal position by sitting directly on your seat bones, and stretch both arms up into a streamlined position. By gently squeezing your gluteal (bottom) muscles, start to bounce on the ball, making sure that the spine maintains its neutral curve. As you become more proficient, increase the size of the bounce.

To increase the effect of the exercise, add alternate side arm movements as you bounce (see page 32).

Creating a Programme

If you have performed them well, the above exercises should have taught you to stabilise your trunk as you move your arms and legs. Now it is time to create a core stability programme.

For best results, it is important to structure a core stability programme so that a variety of positions and body parts are emphasised. The next section outlines a collection of exercises that will teach you to activate the major muscle groups involved in core stability. Some of these exercises have progressions – select the most appropriate for your ability level by beginning with the easiest and working towards the level that challenges you. It is important, however, not to progress until an exercise is performed with perfect form, and can be maintained for 10 repetitions. This ensures that you have first developed the coordination necessary to perform an exercise correctly, and then achieved the endurance to sustain it. Once you have developed the basic skills trained by these exercises, you can begin to select other exercises to address your needs.

Unlike other workouts, *The Core Workout* does not designate set numbers of repetitions. This is because there will be individual limitations and differences, and where some exercises may be easy, others will be more challenging. If you try to perform too many repetitions of a challenging exercise, you may lose your form, and no further benefit will be gained once this happens. As a guideline, aim to perform 3–4 sets of between 4–10 repetitions.

As previously mentioned, if 10 can be performed well, you have the option to progress the exercise if alternatives are offered, or simply increase the repetitions or sets. The exercises are best performed several times per week, to increase coordination and develop form.

To make the most of these exercises, they need to be done with concentration and focus. It is easy to cheat by doing them too fast, and aiming for quantity, not quality. Remember, if it is results that you want, there is no easy path. ***Form is everything***.

Key Elements

As a guide, we have designated a collection of exercises as Key Elements, exercises that provide a foundation around which you can build your programme. These key elements are:

1. Superman

- Four point position
- Applicable for neck, shoulder, lower back and hip work
- Addresses balance of muscles from the upper back down to the hip
- Muscular focus on lower trapezius, lower abdominals, gluteals (bottom muscles)

2. Wall Squat

- Upright position
- Applicable for lower back, hip, groin, knee and ankle work
- Addresses lower power zone, trunk stability and controlled hip bending
- Muscular focus on gluteal muscles, lower abdominals, quadriceps (front of thigh)

3. Wall Push-up

- Upright position
- Applicable for neck, shoulder, elbow, mid and lower back
- Addresses upper power zone and trunk stability
- Muscular focus on lower abdominals, triceps brachii, pectoral muscles, scapular stabilisers (lower trapezius and serratus anterior)

4. Floor Bridge

- Supine (face up) position
- Applicable for spine from neck to lower back, hip, hamstring and knee
- Addresses lower power zone and trunk stability
- Muscular focus on lower abdominals, gluteal muscles, hamstrings

5. Suspension Bridge

- Supine (face up) position
- Applicable for spine from neck to lower back, hip, hamstring and knee
- Addresses lower power zone and trunk stability
- Muscular focus on gluteal muscles and lower abdominals

6. Over the Top

- Prone (face down) position
- Applicable for neck, shoulder, elbow, mid and lower back
- Addresses upper power zone and trunk stability
- Muscular focus on shoulder muscles, midback and lower abdominals

This combination targets the major positions, movements and muscle groups and provides a well-rounded starter programme. These are Level 1 exercises, but depending upon your ability, you may need to begin with a level higher. For example, you may find the Wall Squat quite easy, so you may elect to progress to a higher level of this exercise. You are still working with a Key Element, but at the level appropriate for you. You can then build around the Key Elements by adding exercises which appeal to you, or which address your needs. Try to select exercises in a variety of positions, as these will work different muscle combinations. Examples of a Level 1 programme may be:

1. Key Elements 1, 3, 4, 6 ✛ Seated Leg Raise

2. Key Elements 2, 3, 5, 6 ✛ Neutral Bounce With Arm Movement ✛ Titanic

These combinations targets the major positions, movements and muscle groups and provide a well-rounded starter programme.

1. Superman

This exercise is a multipurpose manoeuvre, coordinating the whole trunk and teaching sound movement principles. The components can be done alone or in combination.

Level 1. Learning shoulder-blade control

Lie over the ball on all fours. Your hands may most comfortably touch the floor on the side of the ball, rather than in front of the ball. Stabilise the trunk by scooping the stomach, and make sure that your head and neck are in a straight line from the shoulders. It is common in this movement to let the head sag down towards the floor, or to tilt the head up and back which overuses the neck muscles. This will lead to poor movement quality.

Now raise an arm straight in front of you. For best quality, imagine that the arm is being lifted gently from the fingers. As your arm rises, visualise your shoulder-blades sliding flat down your rib cage towards your toes. You may find that because of tight muscles you will reach a limit in how far you can lift without your shoulder-blades moving up towards your ears. If this is the case, only move as far as you can with good control. Sustain the position for the count of 5, and then repeat with the other side.

START POSITION FOR SUPERMAN

LEVEL 1: STRAIGHT ARM POSITION WITH
SHOULDER-BLADE CONTROL

Level 2. Learning pelvic girdle control

Lie over the ball on all fours. Lengthen the back of the neck and draw the tummy up to stabilise the trunk as in step one, then slowly straighten one leg out by pressing through the heel, keeping the toe close to the floor in the initial stages. Use your bottom muscles to create the movement, and to prevent the supporting hip from sagging sideways.

Your finish position should achieve a straight line from ears to heel. The foot should not be above the level of the hip, as this would indicate excessive back muscle activity. You are aiming to keep your hips level and trunk stable, and straighten your hip without causing the lower back to arch.

LEVEL 2: STRAIGHT LEG POSITION WITH PELVIC GIRDLE CONTROL

Level 3. Putting it together

Now try combining the two movements together, stretching out with opposite arm and leg.

LEVEL 3: OPPOSITE ARM AND LEG EXTENDED

Level 4. Strong and balanced

Assume a position over the ball where one leg is extended without overusing the back, and you are not using the arms to balance. Begin with one arm up and the other by your side.

Maintaining your trunk position, alternate arms back and forth. After 4–5 repetitions, swap legs. Progress to stretching both arms out in front of you with one leg extended. After a count of 5, replace the extended leg and extend the other leg. You may also progress to rising up on to your toe.

LEVEL 4

LEVEL 4: BOTH ARMS EXTENDED

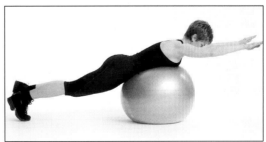

LEVEL 4: BOTH ARMS EXTENDED AND BALANCING ON YOUR TOE

2. Wall Squat

This exercise improves your spinal awareness, increases hip stability and teaches you to balance the forces across your pelvis. It strengthens the thighs and buttocks. Athletes with poor core stability will tend to overuse their inner thighs and lower back.

Stand with the ball in the curve of your back against the wall. Feet should be shoulder-width apart, stomach scooped, bottom lightly squeezing.

Look straight ahead

Keep your shoulders relaxed

Gently scoop your stomach

Knees in line with hips and ankles

Feet shoulder-width apart

START POSITION FOR
WALL SQUAT

1. Slowly roll down the wall to a point that is no further than 90 degrees at the knee.
2. Hold the position for 10 seconds. Roll back up the ball.

Common Errors for the Wall Squat

The trunk should remain vertical, with hips and shoulders in line. Two main errors occur:

1. Failure to flex the hips
2. Sneaking the bottom under the ball

If you can perform a good controlled Wall Squat, you may progress in a variety of ways.

Progression 1. Single heel lift
Lift one heel and then perform the squat. This will demand slightly more effort from the other leg.

Progression 2. Ski shift
Squat to a comfortable depth. Keeping shoulders and hips in line, move across the ball to one side. Make sure that the hips and shoulders do not lose their alignment.

Progression 3. Cross body lift
Start in standing with the ball behind you and a small weight positioned at the left hip. As you squat down, lift the weight across your body towards the opposite shoulder. As you move back up, let the weight lower to its start point at the hip. Keep the pelvis level and the hips and knees pointing straight ahead. The hips should not move out to the side as the weight crosses the body!

3. Wall Push-up

Level 1

A Wall Push-up can be unexpectedly challenging if performed correctly, and is recommended as a start point for developing good push-up form. It is particularly useful if recovering from a shoulder injury, beginning to develop upper limb/trunk coordination, or learning to maintain a neutral spine position.

The degree of difficulty is dictated by the distance of your feet from the ball.

START POSITION FOR THE WALL PUSH-UP

- Start standing upright with your elbows slightly bent. This will be the easiest position from which to control your spine. As you improve, you may start with your feet further from the wall, so that your trunk begins on a slight forward tilt. This would be increasing the lever in order to progress, as shown in level 1+.

- Draw yourself upwards and lengthen through the back of the neck, feeling the abdominals automatically draw inwards. Relax your shoulders so that your push will come from your upper power zone.

LEVEL 1: BENT ELBOW POSITION FOR THE WALL PUSH-UP

The only joints that will move are your elbows. Your spine will stay exactly the same shape throughout the movement. It will not sag or bend at any point. This control comes from your lower abdominals. Which will remain drawn in throughout the movement.

- As your elbows bend, imagine the force travelling from your elbows into your midback. When pushing out, visualise the pushing force coming from the stomach to cue your hips to stay in line with your shoulders.

POOR SCAPULA POSITION FOR THE WALL PUSH-UP

Level 1+

To slightly increase the difficulty of the Wall Push-up, narrow the base by bringing the feet together.

To further increase the difficulty, lengthen the lever by slightly moving your feet further away from the wall.

To increase rotational control, shorten the lever by stepping in again, and lift your body up to place it on one leg, making sure that the hips remain parallel to the wall at all times through the motion.

Order of Progression

The push-up movement is a very versatile exercise, which can be used to target different body parts and functions. You are advised to follow the following progression with the push-up exercises.

Level 1
Wall Push-up

Level 2
Floor Push-up

Level 2
Single Arm Wall Push-up

Level 3
Full Body Push-up

A Note on Breathing

It is common during these higher levels of the push-up for athletes to hold their breath. This is not safe or effective practice. Instead, it is advisable to breathe normally throughout the excercise. You may need to count out loud or whistle as you perform the movement. This helps to maintain your breathing cycle and facilitate an abdominal contraction, which is essential for correct performance of the push-up.

Level 2. Single Arm Wall Push-up

This is a challenging exercise for athletes of any level. Assume a starting position as for the Wall Push-up. Release one hand, and support the arm to be exercised by lowering the shoulder-blade and flattening it into the rib cage.

The movement principles are the same as for the Wall Push-up; however now you must concentrate on keeping your shoulders and hips parallel with the wall.

LEVEL 2: SINGLE ARM WALL PUSH-UP

POOR SCAPULA AND TRUNK POSITION

Level 2. The Floor Push-up

This exercise coordinates the trunk with the shoulder girdle. It strengthens chest, triceps and abdominal muscles.

Place the ball against the wall, and kneel in front of it with your hands comfortably apart.

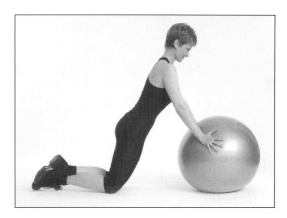

LEVEL 2: START POSITION FOR THE
FLOOR PUSH-UP

Keep shoulders relaxed away from your ears, and maintain an open chest

Control spine by drawing in abdominals

Resist the urge to poke chin

LEVEL 2: FINISH POSITION FOR THE
FLOOR PUSH-UP

Level 2+

The Floor Push-up can be made more difficult by moving the ball away from the wall.

Progress to a Full Body Push-up (see page 52).

Level 3. Full Body Push-up

Perform the exercise in full push-up position. This will demand a great deal of abdominal control. Make sure that you can achieve a controlled movement with the ball against the wall before trying the exercise without wall support.

Scoop the abdominals up towards the spine, straighten your hips and keep your shoulders away from your ears to maintain alignment.

LEVEL 3: FULL BODY PUSH-UP START POSITION

LEVEL 3: FULL BODY PUSH-UP

LEVEL 4: FULL BODY PUSH-UP WITH
FEET ELEVATED

4. Floor Bridge

Level 1. Straight Leg Bridge

This exercise promotes coordinated activation from the buttock muscles in conjunction with a balanced, stable trunk.

To perform a Straight Leg Bridge, start with the ball under your legs and close to your body. By pressing out and down into the ball with the backs of your legs, roll yourself up off the floor until your hips and knees are straight. For extra emphasis, pull your toes back towards you so that your ankles are bent.

START POSITION FOR LEVEL 1 STRAIGHT LEG BRIDGE WITH ARMS ON FLOOR

LEVEL 1+: STRAIGHT LEG BRIDGE WITH ARMS ACROSS CHEST

Once you can balance in this position, progress to placing your arms across your chest as you perform the movement, which will decrease your base of support and increase the stability challenge.

To progress further, start with both arms up to the ceiling, perform the Bridging movement, and then move one arm out to the side. Bring it back to the centre and repeat with the other side.

LEVEL 2: STRAIGHT LEG BRIDGE WITH ARM MOVEMENT

Floor Bridge Adaptations

The bridging exercise can be modified to achieve slightly different effects.

Level 2. Bent Knee Bridge

This exercise trains buttock and hamstring *strength* as well as trunk stability. If you want to focus on your glutes, perform the exercise with the ball close to your hips. If you wish to focus more on hamstrings, start with the ball slightly further out. Lie on your back with your feet on the ball. Initially, use your elbows for support if necessary. Scoop your stomach up and in and check that your neck is relaxed.

Tighten your glutes and slowly peel your hips from the floor by pressing down on the ball. It is important to visualise pushing down through your feet, to help to focus your effort into your legs rather than your back. Aim to keep your back relatively relaxed while working hard on your buttocks and legs. To do this, you may need to tip your pelvis back slightly towards you which will help to counteract a common tendency towards back arching. If you are an athlete, you may eventually find it appropriate to move onto higher levels of these exercises, as follows.

LEVEL 2: BENT KNEE BRIDGE WITH ARMS ABOVE

LEVEL 2: BENT KNEE BRIDGE WITH ARM TO SIDE

Level 3. Straight Single Leg Bridge

Perform the Straight Leg Bridge with both arms on the floor to increase your base of support. Once you have your balance, lift one leg off the ball, keeping your trunk and pelvis level.

LEVEL 3: STRAIGHT SINGLE LEG BRIDGE

Level 3. Bent Single Leg Bridge

Begin with both feet on the ball, and perform the Bent Knee Bridge. When balanced, straighten one knee.

LEVEL 3: BENT SINGLE LEG BRIDGE

5. Suspension Bridge

This exercise trains your gluteal muscles to work with your abdominals to control your trunk and pelvis. Take up a position where your head and shoulders are resting on the ball, and your stomach 'scooped' in.

LEVEL 1: SUSPENSION BRIDGE POSITION

Check your neck alignment, and that your back is not arching. Feel your back muscles: if they are rigid, soften your hips a little and tip your pelvis back towards you. Re-check your back muscles. They should be a little less obvious and your gluteal muscles should feel as though they are working more effectively.

Level 1

Reach your arms up towards the ceiling and slowly move one arm out to the side. Although your body may feel as though it wants to rotate towards the arm, keep it straight and level. This trains rotational stability in the trunk and pelvis. Slowly bring the arm back to the start position and repeat with the other arm (not illustrated). If you can perform this movement well, you may progress to **Level 2**.

Level 2

Keeping your pelvis level and your buttocks squeezing, lift the toes of one foot and the heel of the other. Now swap sides, so that the trunk is in the same position, but the heel/toe lift is opposite. Alternate back and forth for a count of six, and then rest. This equals one set. Aim eventually for ten sets. Remember to keep your pelvis level – we often see the hips sinking slowly towards the floor, which means that your buttocks have switched off! To rest between sets walk back up the ball, e.g. the Walkout (see page 60).

LEVEL 2: SUSPENSION BRIDGE POSITION

6. Over the Top

This exercise builds abdominal control and teaches good alignment. Begin by kneeling behind the ball.

Push out over the ball and support yourself with your hands. The ball should be positioned at mid thigh level. Think long back of the neck, and strong shoulders. Draw your stomach up towards your spine so that the lower back and hips are straight. If you cannot keep this position, roll slightly back onto the ball to decrease the lever. Check your *lower back alignment* – common errors are either to sag, or to pull up with your hip muscles. Instead, imagine a straight line from your ears to your ankles.

START POSITION FOR OVER THE TOP

LEVEL 1: CORRECT OVER THE TOP POSITION

INCORRECT OVER THE TOP POSITION
(PULLING UP WITH HIPS)

INCORRECT OVER THE TOP POSITION (SAG)

Once you have established the basic position, push with your arms so that the body moves back on the ball, keeping a straight body line. Then pull with the arms so that the body moves forwards over the ball, keeping a straight body line. Your trunk should not sag or bend in the middle – try to maintain a long, straight shape throughout the movement. Repeat four times to create a set. Once you can keep the correct balance, use the shoulders and arms to move the body over the ball in a circle. The trunk should stay still, supported by the abdominals, while the shoulders produce the movement. Once again, maintain a strong, straight body line, with no hip or spine movement. Move two circles to the left and two circles to the right to create a set.

LEVEL 2: PUSHING BACKWARDS AND PULLING FORWARDS

Produce the movement from the shoulders, not the spine. The movement is generated from the arms and the trunk does not bend to create the movement.

To progress, start with the ball further down your legs – the further it is from your trunk, the greater the demand on your abdominals. Remember, even if the ball needs to be at the upper thigh level in order for you to achieve good form, you are still gaining benefit.

VIEW FROM ABOVE WHEN CIRCLING LEFT

Library of Exercises

The following exercises can be used to develop your programme. Try to achieve a variety in positions and action as well as working upper and lower body muscle groups.

1. Titanic

Level 2 exercise

Once you have mastered a basic Superman, you can add the Titanic. Its purpose is to strengthen and coordinate the hip extensor and back extensor muscle groups.

Place the ball under your hips, and your feet on the wall near the floor. Allow your body to rest over the ball, so that the hips are slightly bent. Scoop abdominals. Keeping fingertips on the floor, squeeze the hips forwards into the ball, using the glutes strongly. If you feel secure, you can withdraw the fingertips and take your arms to the side, so that you are supporting mainly with your glutes. Do not raise the trunk above the level of the hips, as this will create excessive back extensor muscle activity. Count to 5.

2. Walkout

Level 2 exercise

This exercise takes your body through an arc, which works your abdominals to stabilise and control.

Sit comfortably on the ball with neck and shoulders in neutral. Tuck your chin in and start to walk slowly down and away from the ball, keeping your stomach **scooped in**.

STARTING POSITION FOR
THE WALKOUT

MIDWAY POSITION FOR
THE WALKOUT

Try to keep the **chin in** and the **stomach scooped** until you reach a point where your shoulders are resting on the ball. Relax your back and support yourself using your buttocks. This is the *Suspension Bridge position*, as shown in 'Key Elements' (see page 55).

SUSPENSION BRIDGE POSITION

Begin to walk back up the ball, curling from the chin and keeping the stomach flat.

WALKING UP THE BALL

3. Sway

Level 2 exercise

This exercise trains trunk alignment and hip stability. Walk out into the Suspension Bridge and position your arms horizontally, parallel to the floor. Check that your neck and lower back are neutral (it is easy to slip into back arching) and that your buttocks are working.

Move your legs apart a little further than for the Suspension Bridge.

START POSITION FOR THE SWAY

Keep your trunk and hips in line and without moving your feet, shift over the ball to the left. The ball will roll under your shoulders, towards your right. Feel your weight transfer to your left buttock.

LEVEL 1: SWAY TO THE LEFT SIDE

LEVEL 1: SWAY TO THE RIGHT SIDE

Your legs should remain pointing forwards. If you find your knees moving in the opposite direction to your shoulders, you have released your abdominals! Repeat on the other side.

4. Single Leg Suspension Bridge

Level 3 exercise

Prior to progressing to the Level 3 Suspension Bridge, first gain control and endurance of the **Sway**, which is the previous exercise. Once you are confident and capable with the Sway, you can move onto Suspension Bridge Level 3.

Start with your feet closer together. Focus your mind into whichever buttock is going to support you and slowly peel the other heel off the floor. Scoop the abdominals, and straighten the knee so that you are only supported on one leg. Count to 5, replace the leg and repeat on the other side.

To avoid cheating by arching your back, keep your focus on your supporting buttock as you perform this exercise.

LEVEL 3: SUSPENSION BRIDGE POSITION

Progress to reaching your arms over your head in this position and counting to 5 before swaping sides.

LEVEL 3: SUSPENSION BRIDGE POSITION WITH
EXTENDED LEG

Remember that there is no advantage to performing a more advanced progression if you are unable to maintain neutral in the previous movement.

Level 4

You now have the option of increasing the demands of the exercise by moving your arms or introducing a weight.

LEVEL 4: EXTENDED LEG POSITION WITH
ARM VARIATIONS

LEVEL 4: EXTENDED LEG POSITION WITH
A WEIGHT

5. Ham Sandwich

Level 2 exercise

Begin in the Suspension Bridge position. Keeping your hips level, push with your feet so that your knees straighten slightly.

LEVEL 1: PUSH OUT FOR THE HAM SANDWICH

FINISH POSITION FOR THE HAM SANDWICH

Keeping your hips from sagging towards the floor, pull with your feet until your knees are bent. ***Repeat up to 10 repetitions.***

NOTE: This will seem very easy if you do not concentrate on keeping your hips absolutely level. The focus will be on your abdominals, buttocks, and hamstrings contracting, and the muscles on the tops of your thighs and hips stretching.

When you have mastered the Ham Sandwich, progress to the Level 3 Single Leg Ham Sandwich. This will combine the skill of the advanced Suspension Bridge with extra hamstring and quadriceps effort.

Assume the same start position as for the two leg exercise, and then raise one leg to achieve the advanced Suspension Bridge. Concentrate on keeping your pelvis level. Now pull yourself forwards towards your feet as in the double leg Ham Sandwich.

LEVEL 3: SINGLE LEG HAM SANDWICH

6. Hamstring Pull

Level 3 exercise

This exercise trains buttock strength and provides an intense hamstring workout.

Lie on your back with your feet on the ball. Scoop your stomach, and check neck alignment.

Press down into the ball with your feet and squeeze your buttocks to lift them from the floor. Remember to support this position with the buttocks, not by arching the back.

Consistent buttock activity keeps the hips straight

Keep your back relaxed. If you cannot do this, try tipping your pelvis slightly back towards you

STEP 1: PRESSING DOWN INTO THE BALL

STEP 2: STRAIGHT HIP POSITION IN PREPARATION FOR THE HAMSTRING PULL

Once you can balance in this position, let your feet push the ball out a small distance. You must only push the ball as far as you can without letting your back arch, and no further.

Maintain a neutral spine. If you push out too far, you will arch your back and overuse your back muscles. Check the alignment of your neck and lower back. Now pull the ball back towards you until

STEP 3: PRESSING THE BALL STRAIGHT OUT

you are back to the start position. Repeat the movement at a controlled speed. To make this exercise slightly more difficult, lift your arms up towards the ceiling while performing the movement.

Level 4

When you have mastered the Hamstring Pull, progress to a Single Leg Hamstring Pull. Follow the same guidelines as for the Hamstring Pull. However, because the Single Leg Pull is more difficult, consider reducing your range.

It is vital that you prevent your back from arching by focusing your mind on your buttocks and stomach.

LEVEL 4: FINISH POSITION FOR THE SINGLE LEG HAMSTRING PULL

7. Ball Stability Curl

Using the ball increases abdominal activation in this version of the classic curl-up.

Start with a Suspension Bridge position. Scooping the abdominals down to the spine, breathe out and curl your body as if rolling a wheel down your front. Make sure the lower belly stays pinned down. Keep the muscles working and uncurl again.

8. Around the World

Level 2 exercise

This exercise builds rotational control and strengthens the abdominals and glutes.

Kneel behind the ball. Push forwards so that your hips straighten and the ball supports your chest with your head in a relaxed neutral position. Grasp the ball with your arms.

Excessively using the back muscles and hip flexor muscles to compensate for weak abdominals

START POSITION FOR AROUND THE WORLD

POOR POSTURE DURING AROUND THE WORLD

Keeping the balls of your feet on the floor, slowly roll the ball to one side. Pull back to the centre using the abdominal muscles, squeeze your glutes, and slowly let the ball roll to other side.

FRONT VIEW OF START POSITION

ROLLING TO THE RIGHT DURING AROUND THE WORLD

9. Pendulum Roll

Level 3 exercise

Begin in a Suspension Bridge position with your arms towards the ceiling. Slowly roll your shoulders and arms to one side, allowing the ball to roll slightly in the opposite direction.

Concentrate on keeping your pelvis level as your arms move. You will need to stay focused on the glutes pushing up firmly on the side towards which your arms are moving. Using control from the abdominals, slowly rotate in the other direction.

You may progress to using a weight to increase the demands of the Pendulum Roll. Remember however, that even a very light weight can greatly increase the intensity of this exercise.

START POSITION FOR THE
PENDULUM ROLL

PENDULUM ROLL TO THE
RIGHT

PENDULUM ROLL TO THE LEFT

PENDULUM ROLL WITH A WEIGHT
(START POSITION)

PENDULUM RIGHT WITH A WEIGHT

10. Arm Stabiliser

Level 3 exercise

The Arm Stabiliser builds stability in the arms and shoulders. For safety, perform this exercise with the ball against the wall. Pressing the ball firmly into the wall with your legs, push down with your hands and lift your hips slightly forwards. Moving only a few centimetres to start with, press the ball slightly to the left, and then to the right.

Keep your body straight and still as you move your arms to the right

START POSITION FOR THE ARM STABILISER

MOVING THE BALL TO THE LEFT DURING THE ARM STABILISER

MOVING THE BALL TO THE RIGHT DURING THE ARM STABILISER

When you have gained confidence and skill, you can perform it a small distance from the wall.

11. Tricep Test

Level 3 exercise
Initially, perform this exercise with the ball in a corner for increased safety and stability. When you have gained confidence and skill, you can move the ball slightly away from the wall.

Maintaining an open chest, allow the elbows to bend (dip) to a controllable angle, and squeeze them straight again to re-assume the starting position. Repeat. The number of repetitions depends upon your ability to maintain an excellent shoulder position.

Minimize the distance you need to move forwards; you should only just clear the ball

TRICEP TEST START POSITION

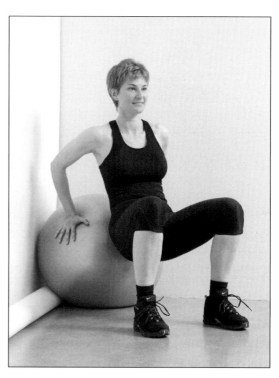

TRICEP TEST FINISH POSITION

12. Windmill

Level 2+ exercise

The Windmill teaches the gluteal muscles to support the back by controlling your hip angle, and trains the abdominals to both stabilise against, and create rotational movement.

Begin by lying over the ball on your stomach, with your feet on the floor. Scoop your abdominals up towards your spine. In order to level your body, squeeze your gluteal muscles to straighten the hip. Your initial attempt will probably involve trying to use the back muscles to pull your shoulders up; try to relax the back and focus on pulling from the gluteals.

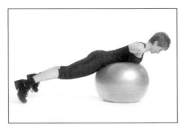
LEVEL 2: START POSITION FOR THE WINDMILL

WINDMILL TURN TO THE LEFT

WINDMILL TURN TO THE RIGHT

Notice that the athlete's back is not straining to lift the shoulders, but is instead maintaining a fairly neutral position with the chest supported by the ball.

Now that you have achieved a reasonable position, turn your upper trunk so that one hand touches the floor. Your hips should stay relatively level. Return to the start position. Tilt your upper body in the other direction.

Alternative

The exercise can also be performed with your feet supported on the wall. As with the floor-based Windmill, turn your upper trunk so that one hand touches the floor.

START POSITION FOR THE WALL WINDMILL

WINDMILL POSITION TO THE LEFT

WINDMILL POSITION TO THE RIGHT

Now return to the start position and rotate to the other side.

13. Body Spin

Level 3 exercise

The Body Spin requires multiple actions of the abdominal muscles. They must control the back angle, and also control rotational movement.

Begin by lying over the ball on your lower ribs, with your feet on the floor or supported by a wall. Scoop your abdominals up towards your spine. In order to level your body, squeeze your gluteal muscles to straighten the hip.

Your arms are out in front of you and your spine should be neutral.

START POSITION FOR THE BODY SPIN

Slowly turn your hips to one side, allowing your feet to release and face the direction in which you are moving. Try not to let your body bend at the waist.

Slowly turn back to the starting position, feeling the focus in your abdominals as they control your speed. Repeat to the other side.

FINISH POSITION FOR THE BODY SPIN

FINISH POSITION FOR THE BODY SPIN
(OPPOSITE DIRECTION)

14. Ramp

Level 3 exercise

This exercise demands abdominal support, upper body strength and shoulder stability.

Address the ball as you would for the Push-up, with the body straight, stomach scooped, the head in neutral and the shoulder-blades away from the ears and flat on the rib cage. Support your weight through your arms.

LEVEL 3: START POSITION

LEVEL 3: MOVING THE BALL AWAY FROM THE BODY

Now move the ball slightly to one side, maintaining a neutral back angle. Move it to the other side, up, back or around in a circular motion to work the shoulders in different positions. You should also feel quite a burn in the abdominals if you are doing this properly!

- Do not allow your back to sag
- Keep your hips straight
- Do not allow your shoulders to creep up to your ears

LEVEL 4: LONG LEVER RAMP

LEVEL 5: REDUCED BASE LONG LEVER RAMP

15. Ball Squat Thrust

Level 3 exercise

Begin in the Over the Top position. Draw your abdominals up towards your spine and pull the ball towards your body with your lower legs. The body should stay straight as the hips smoothly bend.

START POSITION FOR BALL SQUAT THRUST

MIDDLE POSITION FOR BALL SQUAT THRUST

Maintaining strong shoulders, and supported head and lower back, move the ball back out to the start position. Visualise a long straight line from your ears to your toes, and your abdominals pulled up to make your waist narrow.

BALL SQUAT THRUST FINISH POSITION

To progress, try this with a single leg.

16. Ab Burner

Level 4 exercise

This advanced exercise builds abdominal strength and control. It requires concentration and excellent form.

Kneel behind the ball, with your elbows on the ball. Keeping your stomach scooped and lower back neutral, push the ball away from you a short distance, until there is a straight line from your shoulder to your hips.

START POSITION FOR THE AB BURNER

FINISH POSITION FOR THE AB BURNER

Maintaining alignment, pull the ball back towards you with your elbows, then push it away again. The movement should only occur at the shoulders, not the back.

Progress to a full body Ab Burner. Gradually straighten your body, so that there is a straight line from the back of your head to your knees.

LEVEL 5: PROGRESSION TO FULL BODY AB BURNER START POSITION

Push down strongly into ball

LEVEL 5: EXTENDED ARM POSITION FOR THE AB BURNER

Now move the ball away a short distance with your arms. If your back wants to sag, do not go any further. Maintain the upwards impulse with the lower abdominals towards the spine to maintain alignment, and move the ball back towards you.

Do not push beyond your limits. If you cannot maintain a neutral lower back by scooping your abdominals, you have gone too far. This will not make you stronger or more stable.

17. Caterpillar

Level 4 exercise

Caterpillar incorporates a second ball to introduce two sources of instability. Assume a position where your hands are on one ball and knees on another. Scoop abdominals and try to attain a neutral position for head, shoulders and lower back.

CATERPILLAR

Move the ball from side to side with your knees, and then progress to moving the arms and legs in opposite directions.

Now try pushing the front ball slightly forwards and bring it back then try pushing the back ball away, and bring it back.

You may combine any of these directions, and add ideas of your own, such as arms moving clockwise and knees anti-clockwise.

Skill Builders

Skill builders are exercises that introduce a more dynamic component to your core stability work. Most of the preceding Core Exercises aim to develop primary muscle activation, strength and coordination, and train trunk stability by using forces exerted by your arms and legs under relatively controlled conditions.

Now that you have a grounding in core stability, you can introduce exercises which demand faster reactions, using balance, momentum and ballistic principles to encourage your body to react appropriately to less predictable forces.

1. Mogul Squat

The Mogul Squat introduces greater neuromuscular control once the Wall Squat has been mastered.

Begin in the position for a Wall Squat. Roll down the wall to the halfway point, and with a quick push through your feet, change the angle of your lower legs and knees by lifting and shifting your heels outwards. As you bring your weight back down, let your knees absorb the movement by bending slightly. Try to maintain this control through the knees, rather than letting your hips sag sideways.

Caution: Do not try to keep the feet planted and rotate through the knees because this will cause harmful stress through the knee joint. Most of the foot should lift from the floor when shifting position.

Notice that the ball will rotate as your hips turn slightly to follow your leg. To ensure good form, imagine a line going across the front of your pelvis, parallel to the floor. Keep this line parallel throughout the movement. Loss of neutral would reflect in that line dipping towards the floor on one side.

If you have mastered the Double Mogul Squat, and you can perform a good normal single leg squat, you can progress to a Single Leg Mogul Squat. Remember not to plant your foot and twist through your knee: you must push and lift the foot slightly to be able to turn safely. Also bear in mind that this is a **Level 4 exercise**, so both control and strength are needed.

2. 4-3-2 Point Balance

These are advanced level exercises for balance and control.

Stand behind the ball with knees in contact with the ball and hands resting on it. Rock forwards gently until your feet lift from the ground and gradually tighten your buttocks. When you are balanced, rock slightly from side to side, forwards and back or in small circles, maintaining your neutral posture.

4 POINT BALANCE

- Do not hunch your shoulders
- Scoop your abs in and squeeze your glutes

Focus on avoiding the Common Errors and maintain your posture when moving on the Swiss Ball. When this is easy, raise one hand, so that you are now balancing on three points instead of four.

Once again, attempt to move the ball slightly.

3 POINT BALANCE (ONE ARM)

If you are able to progress, try replacing your arm and extend one leg.

- Do not arch your back
- Tuck your chin in

Place particular emphasis on squeezing the buttock of the leg you have extended. Once you are comfortable with 3 Point Balance, 2 Point Balance can be attempted by lifting the opposite arm and leg. However, **this is a very unstable position**, and should be approached with caution and care to prevent falling. If your balance is not secure, or if you are at risk if you fall, e.g. you have decreased bone density, or joint instability, do not choose this exercise. 2 Point Balance is actually more difficult than kneeling on the ball.

3 POINT BALANCE (ONE LEG)

2 POINT BALANCE (ONE ARM, ONE LEG)

3. Balance Challenge

Stand behind the ball with the knees in contact and the hands resting on the ball. Rock forwards until your feet are off the ground, and gradually tighten your buttocks. Slowly shift the weight off your hands, and straighten up your hips by using your buttock muscles.

Avoid using your feet to 'cup' the ball and bring your hips forwards by squeezing your glutes.

If this is easy, try to clap your hands in front and then behind you or above your head and behind your waist. Count your claps or time duration on the ball.

Bring your hips forwards

Squeeze your glutes

BALANCE CHALLENGE

4. Wrestle

This exercise is excellent for developing rotational trunk control, dynamic balance and abdominal strength.

Kneel on the ball facing each other. Join hands, or link forearms so that you have a strong hold on each other. Your task now is to exert enough pressure on your partner to challenge his or her balance, but it is also your responsibility to prevent them from losing their balance completely.

THE WRESTLE

In order to do this you must think about the upper power zones, so that your shoulders are relaxed and the forces on your arms are directed to mid-chest level, and also the lower power zones, so that your glutes stabilise your hips, and your abdominals keep your spine in neutral.

Increase the difficulty with greater rotational force via an Arm Wrestle.

THE ARM WRESTLE

5. Slap Hands on the Ball

This version of the kneeling balance exercise requires faster balance reactions and good reflexes.

Kneel on the ball facing each other. Begin fingertip to fingertip, and then one of you will attempt to quickly slap the other's hand, while he or she tries to avoid being caught. Maintain your neutral alignment as you concentrate on your hands!

SLAP HANDS ON THE BALL

6. Sport Specific Drills

The sport specific drills incorporate hand and eye coordination with balancing on the ball. The following examples relate to the sports of netball and rugby.

Balanced Shoulder Pass
Follow the same guidelines as for the Balance Challenge and adhere to the correct passing and catching technique for netball.

BALANCED SHOULDER PASS

Balanced Lateral Pass
You may apply the same principles for other sports.

BALANCED LATERAL PASS

7. Ballistic Push-ups

These exercises increase the demand on your shoulder and scapular stabilisers, as well as requiring good abdominal holding ability to keep the spine in neutral. They should only be performed after you have mastered the standard push-ups detailed in the Core Exercises.

1. Keep it up!

This exercise introduces a ballistic element to upper body training. Set the ball at shoulder height in a corner. Following the principles of the Wall Push-up (neutral posture with a flat stomach) with particular emphasis on keeping your shoulder-blades low and flat, perform a Single Arm Wall Push-up, and quickly swap hands so that you catch the ball before it falls. Make sure that you generate the outward push from the arm and not by shifting your body weight back from the hips. Your trunk should remain neutral throughout the exercise.

DYNAMIC SINGLE ARM
WALL PUSH-UP

Begin with slow push-ups and a quick change, and gradually increase the speed of your hand changeover. Remember, keep your shoulders and hips parallel to the wall and do not let your back sag. Progress to positioning the ball against a flat wall.

DYNAMIC SINGLE ARM WALL PUSH-UP AGAINST A FLAT WALL

2. Plyo Push-up

Wedge the ball in a corner, and kneel a comfortable distance from it. Before trying this ballistic push-up, perform a normal kneeling push-up as featured on page 51, so that you know that you can control your lumbar spine with your abdominals from that distance.

Keeping your body straight, tip forwards to catch yourself by landing on the ball with both hands, and push yourself up again.

DOUBLE HAND PLYO PUSH-UP

The force should be absorbed through your elbows, and into your 'upper power zone' at mid-chest level, not by letting your shoulders hunch up towards your ears! Repeat. When you have mastered the Double Hand Plyo Push-up on your knees, progress to the Alternate Hand Plyo Push-up. This increases the demand on your shoulder stabilisers, and requires a great deal of trunk stability to maintain a neutral lumbar spine.

ALTERNATE HAND PLYO PUSH-UP

8. Walk the Walk

The movement is similar to the Ball Squat Thrust except that you pull the ball with one leg at a time and walk with your hands. Without your feet touching the ground, attempt to cover a distance while balancing on the ball.

WALK THE WALK START POSITION

Once your legs have flexed to a controlled position, walk with your hands until you reach the start position.

WALK THE WALK LEG MOVEMENT

9. Handspring

This exercise trains dynamic trunk stability, and adds a ballistic component to further challenge the shoulders.

Start by kneeling behind the ball. Activate your abdominals by bringing them up and in, as these will be needed to maintain a neutral spine throughout the movement. Pushing through the legs, 'spring' over the ball until you can catch your body weight with your hands. You are aiming to prevent your lower back from dipping towards the floor, and to keep your shoulder-blades flat on your rib cage.

HANDSPRING START POSITION

The most common errors are shoulder-blades hunching up towards the ears, and the lower back dropping towards the floor. Try to keep your trunk neutral, and absorb the force through your elbows.

When you can perform this exercise well, increase the force with which you push through your legs. This will increase your speed over the ball, and requires a higher level of control from your upper body to control the momentum.

When you are confident performing this exercise, you can progress to springing forwards onto one hand. Remember to begin slowly again – landing on one hand is significantly more difficult than landing on two!

HANDSPRING (ONE ARM LANDING POSITION)

10. Twisting Spring

Using the same principles as for the Handspring, the Twisting Spring introduces an increased demand on the whole body by adding lower body movement.

THE TWISTING SPRING

Start by kneeling behind the ball as with the Handspring (see page 85). This time, after your hands contact the floor, bring both knees up to the side for the last part of the movement. As you move back, push out from the legs and turn your body so that you land straight with both legs together. Repeat to the other side. Once this becomes easy, you can try landing on one hand as you bring your knees up to the opposite side.

11. Sprinter

This exercise was devised when working with sprinters to increase the efficiency of their hip flexion on a stable pelvis and trunk. It is aimed at building a stable anchor for the muscles to pull from, and to decrease ineffective movement patterns.

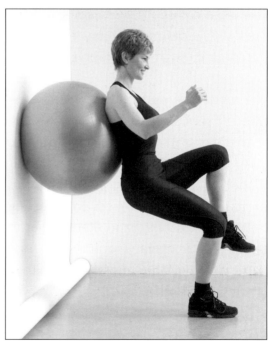

THE SPRINTER

Stand with the ball between you and the wall, and your feet together as you would for the Wall Squat. Activate your abdominals by bringing the stomach up and in, and tighten the glutes of your supporting side.

Keeping the pelvis level and 'open', i.e. facing straight ahead, and your lower back neutral, slowly raise the other knee to a height that you feel that you can control. Control means that you do not let the knee deviate inwards and that you do not 'hip hitch' which avoids using the hip flexor muscles by trying to substitute the muscles on the side of your trunk.

During the movement, your bottom should not sneak under the ball, and your supporting side should not sag. You are aiming for a straight pattern of leg action with minimal trunk or ball movement.

When you have mastered this exercise at a slow speed, begin to introduce the sprinting arm movement and increase your speed of leg movement. Do not be tempted to bend forwards. Keep thinking of being tall and light, and isolating your effort to your lower power zone.

GOOD FORM   POOR FORM   POOR FORM

This is a difficult exercise to perform well, and requires a high level of coordination. The illustrations above show deviations from neutral whereby the athlete is rotating inwards with the right leg and hip hitching. If you are having difficulty performing this movement with the ball, practise with your back directly against a wall, which will provide greater support. **Remember your form!**

12. Pullover

This is a very high level exercise, and requires good coordination, balance and gluteal/abdominal strength. It trains the trunk to remain stable against the resistance of both arms and legs.

Assume a Suspension Bridge position. Lift one foot from the floor and straighten the knee, as for the higher level Suspension Bridge. Extend both arms straight over the head to point at the wall.

Make sure that your pelvis is level, that your stomach is pulled up and in, and that your glutes are working. Bring both arms over the head with the elbows bent, at the same time as bending your hip and knee towards you.

After 4 to 5 repetitions, swap legs.

You will be strongly tempted to let your hips bend so that your bottom sinks towards the floor. Your objective is to maintain a neutral spine, and this will require a great deal of focus on your supporting buttock.

START POSITION FOR THE PULLOVER

THE PULLOVER

INCORRECT PULLOVER

88

13. Kickout

This is also a high-level exercise, which requires a great deal of trunk stability, abdominal strength, coordination and balance.

Stage 1

Prop the ball against a wall, and assume an Ab Burner start position, with your weight directed down through your elbows. Push firmly down into the ball to prevent your shoulders from hunching. Your abdominals should be pulled up towards your spine, and your back in neutral.

THE KICKOUT START POSITION

Without letting this spine position alter, bring one knee up to ninety degrees. Maintaining the spinal position, extend your leg back out to the start position. Repeat 4 to 5 times.

As you improve, you may begin to increase your speed of movement, and if you are very confident, progress to Progression 1 and move the ball away from the wall.

THE KICKOUT WITH WALL SUPPORT

Stage 2

Assume a full Ab Burner position with the ball away from the wall. You are going to perform the same leg movement as for the previous exercise, however this time as your knee moves towards your stomach, you will move the ball in slightly with your elbows.

THE KICKOUT FROM A FULL AB BURNER POSITION

As your leg extends back out, you will move the ball forwards with your elbows. Try to limit the amount of outward movement of the ball to a range that you can control, as illustrated below.

Loss of neutral will often result in back rounding and chin poking.

OUTWARD POSITIONING DURING THE KICKOUT

INCORRECT KICKOUT POSITION

Double Trouble (Partner & Two Ball Exercises)

It can be challenging and fun to work with a partner and/or two balls, and incorporate other factors, such as unpredictability and reaction speed, to further advance your stabilising skills.

A few guidelines must be borne in mind regarding partner and two ball exercises to maximize their benefit, and maintain safety.

Communication

When beginning partner exercises, you will need to let each other know when you are going to move or push, particularly when assuming the start position. Some exercises, e.g. the Double Squat, will need an agreement as to when you will both put full weight against the ball and each other, prior to beginning the movement.

Pacing

When beginning partner exercises, you will need to make direction changes slow and gradual, until you and your partner learn to react with the correct muscles. If you begin with rapid direction changes, and are not adequately prepared or trained, you will tend to activate incorrect muscles, decreasing the effectiveness of the exercise, and increasing the risk of injury. Ideally, you will master unpredictable changes of direction at a slow speed, and gradually increase with practise.

Form

Partner exercises can introduce an element of competition, which can be a positive influence, but is of no use if you sacrifice form for it. Remember that you are working as a two person team aiming for optimal results, and that those results are dependent entirely on the quality of your performance. All the same form tips apply – stomach scooping, neutral alignment, head position and power zones.

1. Standing Double Press

Face each other with the ball at mid-chest height between you. Slowly press into the ball until your arms support your weight.

Perform a push-up against the ball, remembering to maintain neutral alignment from your head through to your lower back. As one partner performs the push-up, the other stabilises. If your coordination as a pair is good, you may both attempt to perform a push-up at the same time.

STANDING DOUBLE PRESS START POSITION

2. Standing Single Arm Press

For much greater neuromuscular challenge, the press can be performed with a single arm. You both must first be able to perform the basic single arm press against the wall before trying this. Face each other with the ball at mid-chest height between you. Initially one person should support the ball with both hands while the other performs the single arm movement.

STANDING SINGLE ARM PRESS START POSITION

Slowly press into the ball until your arm supports your weight. Remember to keep your shoulder-blade flat against your rib cage, and the force directed into your upper power zone. Perform a small elbow bend against the ball, remembering to maintain neutral alignment from your head through to your lower back.

3. Moving Press

This can be done with two hands or one, depending on the level of difficulty required. Face each other with one hand each holding the ball at mid-chest height between you. Designate who will lead the movement first.

Slowly begin to move the ball through a variety of angles, diagonally, up, down, side to side. You may eventually reach a stage where there is no designated leader, and the movement becomes a smooth and fluid exchange between the two of you. This level of fast automatic reaction without effort is an excellent result!

To progress, increase speed, or increase the force exerted through the ball. Do not be tempted to abandon good neutral alignment, because this will decrease your power and control.

To further progress your balance, try using two hands and one foot.

4. Double Pump

Face your training partner with two balls held between you at chest height. Bend your knees slightly to take up a stable position. Make sure that your abdominal and gluteal muscles are working to keep your back and pelvis neutral. Keeping your shoulders down and your necks 'long', both push forwards with your right hand, while letting your left be pushed back. Alternate this movement keeping good form throughout your body.

DOUBLE PUMP ACTION

Once you have achieved a good feel for this movement, gradually increase your pressure on the balls until your arms are working to partially resist the push from your partner. The balls should still move through a full range of motion, but you will need to increase your focus on your power zones to control the forces on your trunk. You will probably have to use more 'abs' and glutes and remind yourself to keep your shoulders down.

When you have achieved good form, you may try to increase your speed.

5. Prone Push-up

Assume a push-up position on opposite sides of the ball. Remember the alignment cues that you have learned from the individual push-up – the same rules apply!

Alternate the push-up, i.e. one holds while the other moves. **Do not forget your form!**

PRONE PUSH-UP

6. Double Ramp

As in the individual Ramp (see page 73) this exercise can be done on knees or feet, depending on your ability.

Hold this position as both players try to move the ball in small degrees in any direction. The challenge is to resist the other player's movement choice.

Do not hold this exercise for too long – this level of stabilising is quite advanced. Thirty seconds is a good starting time.

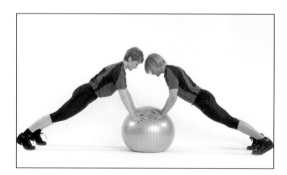

DOUBLE RAMP

7. Double Arm Stabiliser

Refer back to the Arm Stabiliser (see page 69). Assume a position on opposite sides of the ball as pictured.

Each player tries to move the ball a small amount in any direction against the resistance of the other. Be careful to meet and control the resistance offered by your partner, and do not try to push them further than a couple of inches. Do not exceed thirty seconds to begin with.

DOUBLE ARM STABILISER START POSITION

8. Double Dip

Assume a starting position as for the Double Arm Stabiliser and perform alternating dips, i.e. one holds while the other dips.

DOUBLE DIP

9. Double Hip Lift

Lie on your backs with your feet on the ball. Lift the hips by pressing down into the ball with your feet. Remember the form tips from the hamstring pull – stomach scooped, gluteals squeezing, and no back arching. Now try and vary the position of the ball against each other, keeping your pelvis level.

DOUBLE HIP LIFT

10. Single Leg Hip Lift

The aim is the same, i.e. to move the ball in different directions against each other's resistance.

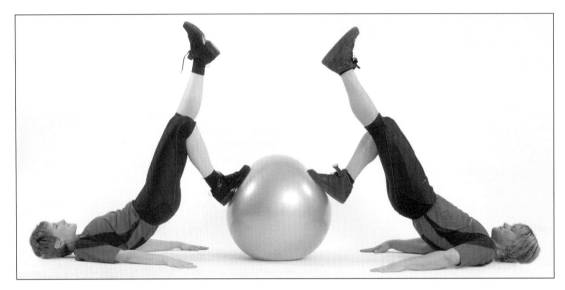

SINGLE LEG HIP LIFT

11. Double Leg Trunk Controller

Lie on your backs with your feet on the ball. Scoop stomachs, and increase the pressure on the ball slightly to raise it off the floor.

DOUBLE LEG TRUNK CONTROLLER

Move the ball against each other in any combination of directions. The aim is to keep the trans abs working (no stomach protruding) and the trunk flat on the floor. If this is too easy, progress to the Single Leg Trunk Controller.

12. Single Leg Trunk Controller

The same principles apply as above, but this time, try controlling the ball with one leg. **Hint: you will need your gluteals to control your hip and leg.**

You will need to concentrate on abdominal scooping and keeping your pelvis flat and level.

SINGLE LEG TRUNK CONTROLLER

Now try it with your opposite feet together. Both legs move independently.

SINGLE LEG WITH FEET TOGETHER

13. Double Leg Squat

The trickiest part of this exercise is balancing your body weights. To do this, you both need to be able to push your backs into the ball at the same time. This can be done even when you have very different body weights, by communicating at the time when you need to push against the other person. This is best done slowly. Your feet will need to start away from the ball so that you can achieve an end position where your knee is no further out than your ankle.

DOUBLE LEG SQUAT

Once you have achieved a balanced starting position, proceed to perform a squat, remembering to use the gluteals to control the movement and the position of the thigh.

14. Single Leg Squat

Try the same exercise, this time with one person bracing while the other performs a Single Leg Squat.

Correct posture

Poor posture

SINGLE LEG SQUAT (ADVANCED)

15. Stacks

These exercises are called 'Stacks' because they involve the ability to withstand an external force, stacked on the ability to control rotation, stacked on the ability to maintain a stable neutral position. They involve two people, and one or two balls. Stacks can be performed in any position relevant to the sport.

Starter Stack

Start in the Wall Squat position, with feet hip-width apart. Bend the knees slightly, draw the abdominals in to support your spine and activate the gluteal muscles to provide a strong lower power zone. Hold the ball at mid-chest level, and open your chest.

STARTER STACK

Your partner will now exert gentle pressure against the ball in different directions.

Suspension Bridge Stack

Follow the principles for the Sway and lie face upwards on a ball in a neutral position. Once again, your partner can exert gentle pressure on the second ball by pushing away, pulling towards, pushing down or pulling up on the ball.

Pushing the ball to the left and right will exert considerable rotational force on your partner while pushing down on the ball stimulates the glutes to work even harder.

Progress to random changes of pressure on the ball – close your eyes and react!

PRESSING DOWN AND SIDEWAYS THROUGH BALL

PUSHING IN ALL DIRECTIONS WITH LONG LEVER

INCREASING TRUNK DEMAND

Ski Stack

Both athletes assume a tuck position with the ball between them. Start to increase pressure through the ball in any combination of directions.

16. Maul

This is a freestanding stack. You now have no external support to depend upon, so you must concentrate on sustaining a stable neutral posture, using the principles of upper and lower body power zones.

As your partner exerts pressure on the ball, you should focus on bringing your stomach towards your spine, keeping your shoulders relaxed, and glutes working. Feel the muscles of your abdominal wall working as you resist the ball pressure.

17. Scrum

This exercise teaches you to use your gluteal and leg muscles to generate forward pressure.

Assume a position in which the ball is resting across the shoulder and upper arm. Find a comfortable position for your feet, and bring your trunk into a neutral position. Bring your stomach in, and focus on pushing through your feet, keeping the pelvis and shoulders pointing straight ahead. Increase the pressure against your partner, and imagine your line of force moving forwards.

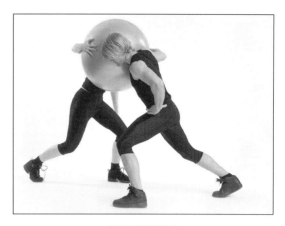

THE SCRUM

18. Linked Sway

Both athletes assume a sway position facing in opposite directions, and link arms. Maintaining a good neutral hip and back position, one athlete will pull against the other, challenging them to activate their abdominals and gluteals to resist the force. Hold for a count of 10 and swap roles.

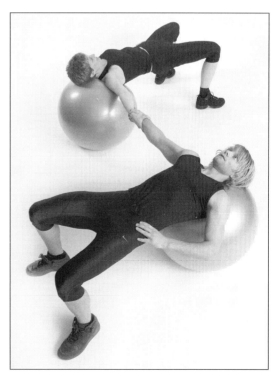

THE LINKED SWAY

Connect Four Exercises

The aim of the 'Connect Four' group of exercises is to introduce push and pull movements from a stable and neutral position with four points on one ball, i.e. two arms and two legs or four arms. An important factor to consider during these exercises is the relative body weights of the partners. As with all Double Trouble exercises, the principles are communication, form and pacing.

19. Push Press

Assume a position where one partner lies on the floor with knees bent, and holds the ball while the other partner begins with the push-up start position.

From the start position, you and your partner have several options. One option is for the upper partner to perform a push-up, relying on the lower partner to stabilise the ball as the force increases during the lowering phase of the push-up. Simply reverse roles to challenge the lower partner to perform a push-up.

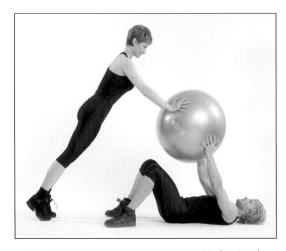

START POSITION FOR PUSH PRESS (FRONT)

UPPER PARTNER PUSH-UP

LOWER PARTNER PUSH-UP

20. Leg Press

One partner now lies on the floor, while the other partner places the ball on his or her feet, and then takes up the push-up position as in the Push Press, with knees and hips straight, stomach pulled up towards the spine, and shoulder-blades on the rib cage.

The floor partner may perform a series of leg presses, concentrating on using the glutes to stabilise the legs. After 5–10 repetitions, the pressing partner may hold a position midway through the leg press range, to allow the other partner to perform push-ups.

Alternatively, this position can be used to let the upper partner perform an individual Ramp (see page 73). Progress to performing these exercises with one leg.

LEG PRESS START POSITION

21. Kneeling Palm Press

Start with the ball at arms length and palms on the ball, making sure that your backs are neutral and the shoulders are down.

Follow the same principles as during the Push Press, and attempt to perform push-ups using the ball as a focal point.

THE KNEELING PALM PRESS START POSITION

THE KNEELING PALM PRESS FINISH POSITION

22. Reactor

This exercise trains quick reactions from your leg, ankle and foot muscles and good body balance.

Sit on the ball with one foot on the ground and a partner holding your other foot. Bring your abdominals up and in.

You are primarily going to work the leg that is linked to the floor. Slightly tighten the muscles of the leg held by your partner so that it can be used to shift your body weight. Your partner will push through your foot to make the ball move forwards and backwards, side to side and at any angle. You will keep your balance on the ball while using your supporting leg to stabilise. Begin slowly in small movements and gradually increase the speed.

Sample Sport Specific Workouts

The following programmes are aimed at guiding you towards core exercises that address elements of a selection of sports. These lists should be regarded as samples only – every individual will have different needs and priorities, and you will find as you work through the book that there are other exercises that may suit your needs. These sample programmes are primarily to help you to problem solve for your sport, whether it is listed or not. By using a range of sports with different demands, we would like to assist you firstly to identify key movement requirements for your sport, and secondly exercises to address them.

In almost all of the sports mentioned, we have observed a strong tendency for the abdominal and gluteal muscles to work inadequately, and for the lower back muscles to work excessively. Many of the athletes who have presented to us with persistent back problems demonstrate this tendency, and it is not only associated with pain, but also loss of muscular efficiency. This should be borne in mind during all of the exercises, and extra care should be given to focusing on the target muscle to be worked, not just 'going through the motions' using old poor muscular habits. If you are unsure how hard your back muscles are working, where possible feel the muscles with your fingers, or ask a training partner to monitor them: if there are big ridges of hard muscle either side of your spine, but your stomach is sagging and your glutes are soft, you know that you are not using the correct proportion of muscular effort. **Remember – form is everything.**

Swimming

Demands of the Sport

- Trunk stabiliser control in a streamlined position
- Balance between hip extensors and back extensors
- Coordinated pattern of upper and lower body stability

Programme

Key exercises
1–6 at the appropriate level for your ability

First level additions
(a) Sway: trains consistent ability to control the trunk position
(b) Wall Squat with arms above head in streamlined position: further trunk control
(c) Titanic: balance and coordination between back and hip extensors

Second level additions
(a) Bodyspin: linear rotational control
(b) Kneeling Press-up: shoulder and trunk support

Double trouble exercises
(a) Standing Double Press
(b) Double Ramp

Best weight training option
Pullover in Suspension Bridge position

Rugby

Demands of the Sport

- Multidirectional control
- Stability against external resistance
- Ability to generate explosive power
- Trunk rotation power and control

Programme

Key exercises
1–6 at the appropriate level for your ability

First level additions
(a) Wall Squat Ski Shift: trains a stable trunk while transferring weight
(b) Pendulum Roll: trains rotational control through the trunk

Second level additions
(a) Caterpillar: multidirectional trunk control
(b) Ab Burner: primary abdominal strength

Skill builders
(a) Balance Challenge: holding a medicine ball, keep your kneeling balance while turning your trunk to move the medicine ball from side to side
(b) Wrestle

Double trouble exercises
(a) Maul
(b) Single Leg Moving Press

Best weight training option
Single leg flyes in Suspension Bridge position

Netball

Demands of the Sport

- Explosive power, forwards and upwards
- Speed with quick acceleration and deceleration
- Agility
- Ability to control rotational forces

Programme

Key exercises
1–6 at the appropriate level for your ability

First level additions
(a) Ham Sandwich: works hamstrings in both a lengthening and shortening action on a stable pelvis to address deceleration
(b) Windmill: trains the glutes to maintain a stable position for the hip and lower back, and the abdominals to create and control trunk rotation for strong accurate passing

Second level additions
Bodyspin: high level rotational control maintaining a neutral spine

Skill builders
(a) Balance Challenge
(b) Slap Hands on the Ball
(c) Sports Specific Drills
(d) Mogul Squat

Double trouble exercises
(a) Double Ramp
(b) Single Leg Hip Lift
(c) Reactor

Best weight training option
Cross Body Pullover, aiming to control trunk rotation through large resisted ranges of motion with the arms

Sprinting

Demands of the Sport

- Ability to maintain pelvic stability against large forces generated by the leg muscles
- Explosive speed
- Sustained efficient linear motion

Programme

Key exercises

1–6 at the appropriate level for your ability. Pay particular attention to attaining high-level progressions in the Superman, to increase the abdominal control of your pelvis and trunk and enhance the activity of your glutes

First level additions

(a) Ham Sandwich: trains pelvis to remain stable while the legs apply stress

(b) Ab Burner: beginning on knees, to train trunk control and high-level abdominal strength

Second level additions

(a) Ball Squat Thrust: trains lumbo-pelvic control against leg movement

(b) Kickout (very high level): integrates the entire body in linear motion with greater strength component

(c) Pullover (very high level): integrates the whole body in linear motion with greater coordination and balance component

Skill builders

(a) Sprinter
(b) Ballistic Push-ups

Double trouble exercises

(a) Single Leg Trunk Controller
(b) Double Pump

Best weight training option

Weighted Wall Squat

Golf

Demands of the Sport

- Ability to sustain a neutral spinal position throughout a large range of motion
- Ability to control rotation throughout the body
- Strong support combined with mobility in the lower limbs

Programme

Key exercises
1–6 at the appropriate level for your ability

First level additions
(a)	Around the World: trains rotational control with a neutral spine position (abdominal bias)
(b)	Pendulum Roll: rotational control with a gluteal bias

Second level additions
(a)	Bodyspin: requires rotational ability with hip mobility
(b)	Windmill: trains rotation of the thorax on a stable lumbo-pelvic region
(c)	Caterpillar: connects upper and lower body through the trunk muscles

Skill builders
(a)	Balance Challenge
(b)	Twisting Spring

Double trouble exercises
(a)	Double Hip Lift
(b)	Stacks
(c)	Maul

Best weight training option
Cross Body Pullover

Demands of the Sport

- Sustained strength from the lower limbs
- Ability to absorb changes in ski angle through lower limbs
- Balance and quick reactions through trunk

Programme

Key exercises
1–6 at the appropriate level for your ability

First level additions
(a)　Sway: trains gluteal endurance and trunk stability
(b)　Hamstring Pull: trains gluteal strength and holding ability and hamstring strength through shortening and lengthening actions

Second level additions
(a)　Caterpillar: whole body stability in a variety of directions
(b)　Ab Burner: advanced abdominal strengthening

Skill builders
(a)　Twisting Spring
(b)　4-3-2 Point Balance
(c)　Mogul Squat

Double trouble exercises
(a)　Stacks
(b)　Leg Press
(c)　Double Leg Squat

Best weight training option
(a)　Weighted Wall Squat
(b)　Cropped Range Lunge

Cricket

Demands of the Sport

- Rotational control
- Speed and agility
- Ability to control large body displacements

Programme

Key exercises
1–6 at the appropriate level for your ability

First level additions
(a) Pendulum Roll: introduces rotational stresses in supine (body facing upwards)
(b) Sway: trains gluteal endurance and trunk stability in lateral movements

Second level additions
(a) Ramp: multidirectional stability for the shoulders arms and trunk
(b) Pullover: very high-level whole body exercise using large range of arm and leg motion
(c) Ball Stability Curl

Skill builders
(a) 4-3-2 Point Balance
(b) Wrestle
(c) Walk the Walk
(d) Slap Hands on the Ball

Double trouble exercises
(a) Stacks
(b) Maul
(c) Standing Single Arm Press

Best weight training option
(a) Batting: Cross Body Pullover
(b) Fast/medium bowling: Outer Range Trunk Lift

Martial Arts

Demands of the Sport

- Ability to maintain a neutral spinal position while rotating the thorax and using arms against resistance
- Ability to retain control in the upper and lower power zones under random conditions (as speed and direction of opponents will vary)
- Ability to control lateral and diagonal movements, maintaining a balanced base

- Ability to control weapons, as the increased leverage of a long weapon elevates the demand for excellent spinal and hip positioning, with gluteal and abdominal muscles providing primary support

Programme

Key exercises
1–6 at the appropriate level for your ability

First level additions
(a) Pendulum Roll: teaches rotational control with gluteal endurance
(b) Single Hand Wall Push-up: teaches scapular control, by learning to focus upper limb effort into the upper power zone

Second level additions
(a) Around The World: trains rotational control with abdominal and gluteal endurance
(b) Ramp: trains trunk and upper limb stability

Skill builders
(a) Balance Challenge
(b) 4-3-2 Point Balance

Double trouble exercises
(a) Moving Press
(b) Stacks
(c) Maul

Best weight training option
Pendulum Roll with one dumbbell

Flexibility Development and Stretching With Your Swiss Ball

The objective of a stretch is to lengthen a muscle. This is important to maintain the range of motion of the joint that the muscle acts upon, to improve the muscle's function, and to prevent injury.

The stretches described in this section should be performed in a smooth, relaxed manner. Resist the urge to 'bounce' at the end of range; this decreases the level of control you have, and tends to make the muscle reflexively shorten.

Each stretch is sustained for the count of 15–30 seconds, and can be performed 2–3 times.

1. Neck Stretch

Sit 'tall' on the ball, with fingertips touching the sides. Without bending at the trunk, slide the fingertips of one hand slightly down the ball, so that one shoulder is slightly lower than the other. Now bend your neck towards the other ear, feeling a gentle stretch down the side of the neck.

Note that the head has not turned, but is looking straight ahead. Hold. Repeat the exercise with the hand reaching down the other side of the ball. Remember, maintain neutral alignment.

To reach muscles further back behind the neck and shoulder, maintain the position of your shoulders and neck, and turn your head to look towards the armpit. Hold. Swap sides.

2. Lat Stretch

Sit 'tall' on the ball, hands over the head, with one hand grasping the wrist of the other. Reach upwards towards the ceiling on the side of the grasped wrist. Now pull the arm to the opposite side, to feel a stretch down the side of the trunk. If you do the upwards reach first, you should not have to bend your trunk much to achieve a stretch. Hold.

3. Tricep Stretch

Sit 'tall' on the ball, and reach with the hand to touch the back of the shoulder of the same side. Make sure that the shoulder itself is relaxed, i.e. not squeezed up towards the ear.

Apply gentle pressure at the elbow with the other hand, in a straight backwards direction. Hold.

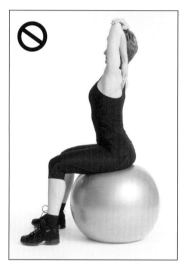

4. Hamstring Stretch

Sit on the ball with one leg slightly bent. Roll the ball backwards, keeping the chest up. Hold.

5. Adductor Stretch

Sit on the ball with one leg out to the side. Roll the ball away from the straight leg, and slightly forwards to feel an inner thigh stretch. Hold.

6. Quad Stretch

Stand on one leg, holding an ankle. Make sure thighs stay together. Draw up the lower abdominals and the gluteal (bottom) muscles, so that the front of the hip straightens. Hold.

Do not let your lower back 'give' into a curve; it makes the stretch less focused, and increases the stress on the lower back.

7. Hip Stretch

Place the ball against the wall, or, for more stability, in a corner. Rest a leg on the ball so that the knee falls outward, and 'sit' in this position.

Keeping the chest up, lean forwards to stretch the hip. Hold.

8. Side Stretch

Kneel side-on to the ball. Straightening the outer leg and reaching with the uppermost arm, stretch across the ball sideways until you find the position that suits you best. You may find that straightening the inner leg stretches more effectively. Hold.

FULL SIDE STRETCH

9. Pectoral Stretch

On hands and knees, rest one forearm on the ball so that the angle of your shoulder is about 90 degrees to your trunk. Turn your head away from the ball so that the chest faces slightly away from the ball. At this point you should feel a stretch across your chest.

Keeping the chest facing away from the ball, roll it slightly upwards away from the body, so that your upper arm is slightly closer to your head. Find the position which best stretches you, and hold.

10. Crossed Arm Stretch

Kneel behind the ball with hands crossed on the top of the ball. Sit back onto your feet so that your arms are now outstretched.

Roll the ball to one side until a stretch is felt under the upper arm and side of the trunk.

Repeat the stretch to the other side.

CROSSED ARM STRETCH TO THE RIGHT

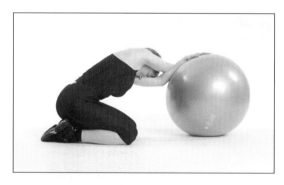

11. Extension Stretch

CROSSED ARM STRETCH TO THE LEFT

Gently lie down on the ball, allowing your spine to relax over the curve of the ball. Breathe normally.

For slightly greater stretch, take both arms over the head.

EXTENSION STRETCH

12. Calf Stretch

There are two main muscles to be stretched in the calf, but rarely does anyone stretch both. Because these muscles influence the knee and ankle in different ways, both should be stretched independently, as set out below.

Stand with one foot fully on a step and the other with only the balls of the feet on the step. Keeping the head and shoulders directly above the hips, and the back knee straight, sink the heel gently downwards. Hold. Sustaining the same position, now slightly bend the back knee. The stretch should feel duller, and closer to the ankle. Hold.

Alternatively, stand with hands against a wall, one foot in front of the other. Keeping your body in line as above, and back knee straight, lean forwards onto front foot.

To stretch the deeper portion of the calf, shift your weight onto the back leg and bend your knee. The pulling is usually duller, and closer towards the ankles.

13. Hip Flexor

Assume a position where the leg to be stretched is in a kneeling position. A pillow or rolled sweatshirt will make this more comfortable for the knee cap. Align head, shoulders and pelvis, and make sure you are not tipping forwards at the waist.

Now draw your abdominals in and tip your pelvis backwards, so that the pubic bone lifts and you feel like you are 'tucking your tail under'. Feel a stretch down the front of the hip and thigh. You may even feel some stretch down the outside of the thigh. Count to 20 and repeat.

 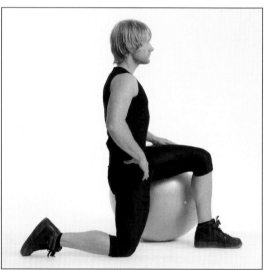

14. Lower Back Warm-up

Sit on the ball with both feet on the floor. Slowly move the ball in a small circle, and gradually make that circle larger. After several repetitions, change direction.

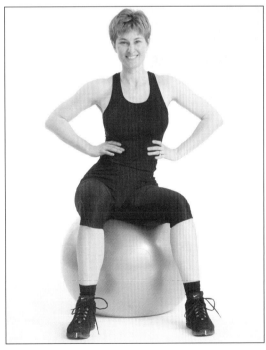

Before the Event

Elements of *The Core Workout* can be very beneficial as part of a pre-game or pre-event warm-up. Optimal performance is dependent on the body's neuromuscular system being primed, and a brief period of demand on an unstable apparatus such as the exercise ball can effectively facilitate this. It is best incorporated after the basic warm-up and stretches have been done, and should take no longer than 5–7 minutes. The exercises should be done with excellent form, and must be done with the aim of stimulating muscular firing. They must not be performed to fatigue.

The recommended individual pre-event exercises are:

- An appropriate level of Balance Challenge to 'wake up' your system
- Sway
- Over the Top
- Handspring

Weight Training With Your Swiss Ball

Throughout *The Core Workout*, we have used the Swiss Ball as the primary tool for stability training. It can, however, be used to complement other forms of training, such as working with weights, and this concept is gaining popularity amongst trainers and sportspeople. For this reason, we will briefly discuss the use of exercise balls in weight training to introduce you to how they may be utilised in your programme. However, it is not the objective of this manual to focus on weight training, and we therefore stress that this is simply an introduction.

Why use exercise balls for weight training?

There are several advantages to using the ball when weight training. One is the ability to make subtle changes to the angle of your effort when lifting. This may allow you to target the range in which you need to work your muscles most. Another is that you can monitor how effectively your body can control a moving weight, as loss of control and compensatory trunk movements will reflect in ball movement. Finally, using the ball while lifting weights stimulates your stabilising muscles to react to limb loading, which increases functional carryover from training into sports.

How do I incorporate the ball into weight training?

Firstly, the principles that you have learned throughout *The Core Workout* will have laid good foundations for your weight training. The concepts of neutral alignment, stomach scooping, breathing and power zones should apply in the same ways to weight training as for core stability work, and often injuries or poor outcomes are results of being unaware of their importance. Remember that you are aiming for the most efficient, most effective and safest methods of training to gain optimal results.

The next thing to bear in mind is that weight training with good form on the ball increases the demand on your neuromuscular system, due to the increased activity required of your stabilising muscles. You will find that your ability to maintain excellent form is dependent on your level of fatigue, and that you may initially fatigue more quickly due to the higher general muscular activity and concentration required to perform the exercises correctly. Adequate recovery time is therefore necessary between sets, as fatigue and decreased coordination are closely correlated, and will lead to compensatory strategies from the body and a loss of efficiency. You may find that your neuromuscular endurance varies from session to session, but by monitoring your body's response and adjusting your rest periods accordingly you will make the most of your effort. Remember: Form is Everything.

Training for optimal muscular activity in this manner has excellent potential for carryover into sporting activity, as performance on the field, track or court is highly dependent on endurance not only of single groups of muscles, but also of the body's ability to repeatedly reproduce a set of skills which depend on complex muscular interactions over time.

When beginning to work with the ball, it is advisable that you use a lower load, higher repetition strategy. It takes practise to adjust to the relative instability of the ball as a support surface, and you need to give yourself time to learn the new muscular patterns that will be necessary. This will be safer if you use a less heavy weight. For this reason, we suggest that you introduce only a couple of exercises using the ball at a time, so that it does not disrupt your regular programme too much, or tempt you to try weights that you cannot control adequately.

Two or three Core Exercises performed during a warm-up can help to stimulate the body's neuromuscular system prior to a workout, but these must not be done to fatigue. The idea is to prime the body for exercise, not put it at a disadvantage by tiring the mechanisms which will make your workout more effective. For similar reasons, after a warm-up the most challenging exercises should be performed first while fatigue has less influence, and less demanding exercises performed as the programme progresses.

Safety Tips

- Do not use foot weights during any of the exercises. You are trying to train your trunk stabilisers to act as your 'anchor', and fixed feet will stimulate the wrong muscle pattern

- Always use a spotter, particularly during movements such as incline bench press where the ball may slip backwards. You may also use a wall to support the ball

- Select lighter weights when using the ball due to the increased neuromuscular demand and increased whole body muscle activity

Examples of Ball Use for Weight Training

The ball can be used as an alternative multi-angled bench

The Bench Press

Those who perform this exercise regularly often try to vary the angle of effort in order to work slightly different parts of the chest muscle and anterior shoulder. Conventional benches can limit the potential for this, but the ball allows very subtle variations.

Notice that the skills that you learned in the Suspension Bridge are necessary here. Abdominals and gluteals need to work, and special attention must be paid to not using the lower back muscles for support. If this is difficult, try tipping the pelvis slightly back towards you.

When varying the angle of effort, be careful to keep the neck and lower back in neutral.

It is vital that you use a spotter during all exercises, particularly when using the ball as a bench. If you do not have a spotter when working on an angle, you may wish to use a wall to support the ball and prevent it from shooting out from under you.

STANDARD BENCH PRESS ON THE BALL

INCLINE BENCH PRESS ON THE BALL

The same idea can be applied to bias muscle groups in slightly different ways. For example, the Suspension Bridge position is used to work latissimus dorsi and long head of triceps brachii, and with a shift of position, triceps brachii and deltoid (shoulder) muscles are working. In this way the triceps group has been worked fully in terms of range, action, and its role in terms of its functional relationship with other muscle groups.

START POSITION   FINISH POSITION

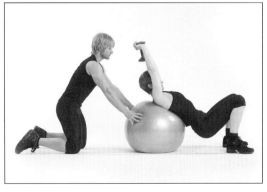

ALTERNATIVE START POSITION   FINISH POSITION

An alternative way to use the ball is for monitoring body balance, incorrect use of momentum, and compensatory body sway

Bicep Curl

Sit on the ball, as you would on a bench in standard dumbbell curls. Begin by lengthening your spine from the back part of the top of your head, allowing your stomach to fall in and your shoulders to settle down and back. Stabilise your scapula by flattening it onto your rib cage, and keep it from rolling up and forwards.

BICEP CURL WITH VERTICAL TRUNK CONTROL

LOSS OF TRUNK POSITION

Now proceed with the bicep curl, but use your abdominal muscles to limit the amount that your trunk moves on the ball. You are aiming for almost no ball movement. The same principle applies to the vertical and lateral raise.

VERTICAL RAISE ON THE BALL

LATERAL RAISE ON THE BALL

Cross-body Patterns With Resistance

It is important to practice this movement without a weight initially, so that you become familiar with the muscle patterns necessary to control the rotational movement, and when introducing weight, to begin with very small amounts. For example, when we introduced this exercise to a group of international rugby players in their late teens, a weight of 2 kgs was more than sufficient to work them hard. You may need to start with as little as 500 grams in some cases – remember that this exercise demands that the trunk and arms control large ranges of motion, and small weights can generate large forces at the extremes of range.

Assume a Suspension Bridge position. Scoop your stomach by pulling up and in with the abdominal muscles, and make sure your buttocks are working to support you. If you feel that your lower back is working more than your glutes, lower your hips slightly and tip your pelvis back towards you to relax the back muscles. The hips must remain level at all times during the motion, and the head and neck in neutral. Try to visualise keeping a 'long neck'.

Grasping the weight in both hands, begin with the arms straight up towards the ceiling. Keeping firm control with your abdominals, move the weight slightly to one side and above your head, in a slow arc. Your trunk will want to arch upwards and twist but your abdominal muscles must control this.

When you reach a comfortable limit with your arms, stabilise firmly with the abdominals and bring the weight slowly over to the hips on the opposite side of your body. Repeat 4–10 times, and then repeat the movement beginning on the opposite side.

CROSS-BODY MOVEMENT TO THE LEFT

CROSS-BODY MOVEMENT TO THE RIGHT

You may use the ball to introduce a balance component to a weights exercise

Wall Ball Squat

Using either a barbell across the shoulders or dumbbells in your hands, you are able to add resistance to the basic wall squat.

Assume a position as for the Wall Squat. Make sure that your feet are far enough forwards to prevent your knee from moving beyond them at the lowest point in your squat. Focus on keeping your spine in a neutral position by scooping your abdominals up and in, and generate support for your pelvis by squeezing your glutes. Keeping the knees in line with the ankles, slowly roll down, to a point where your knees make an angle no less than 90 degrees. Keeping the stomach in, push up again slowly, focusing on pushing from the glutes.

WALL BALL SQUAT WITH DUMBBELLS

You also have the option of raising the dumbbells to shoulder height, and with a barbell, positioning the load in front (front squat position) or behind you (back squat).

Cropped Range Lunge

Start with the ball against the wall and one foot on the ball. Using a low weight at either waist or shoulder height, bend the front knee through a range of motion that can be controlled with the foot flat and the body in neutral alignment. To perform this exercise well, you will need good abdominal support and well activated gluteals.

You can increase the demands of this exercise by using the ball off the wall. Furthermore, some people prefer to move the ball slightly back as they lunge, and bring the ball back to the start position between each repetition.

START POSITION

The ball can also be used for prone support, to make some standard exercises much safer

Reverse Flye

In the reverse flye, it is common to assume a start position that puts the back in a relatively unsafe posture. By using the ball, your chest is supported, taking the strain off the lower back and focusing your efforts into your midback, as is the intended purpose of the exercise. Remember that the same guidelines apply as for every other exercise – abdominals gently scooped, neck in neutral, and shoulder-blades away from the ears and flat on the rib cage.

Superman

Similarly, the same technique can be used for the lower trapezius, but it must be stressed that you should be able to perform the Superman exercise well before weight is applied to the movement. The most common error is to let the shoulder-blade creep up towards your ear as your arm rises.

The ball can be used to exercise through greater ranges of movement

For most of us, the abdominals are more than adequately trained in relatively small ranges of movement. As we have explored throughout *The Core Workout*, the deep muscles of the abdominal wall that are responsible for stability are those most often missed in training, and it is these that we have fundamentally concentrated on.

For some athletes, however, the abdominals responsible for movement play a crucial role in their sport, and in much more vulnerable and demanding positions. For example javelin throwers, fast bowlers and gymnasts need to be able to use the different actions of the abdominal muscles to superimpose a movement role over a stabilising role. For athletes such as these, the ball is ideal to reproduce positions of vulnerability and allow quite specific training. To perform such a movement, the trans abs must be activated first, pulling the stomach in towards the spine, and as the trunk curls up, the focus must be on keeping the stomach gently scooped.

Outer Range Trunk Lift

This is a high-level abdominal exercise, and is only recommended for well-conditioned athletes for whom outer range abdominal control is relevant. It is essential that you have developed good strength and stability in your trans abs by practising a range of the core exercises such as Over the Top, the Ab Burner and Body Spin prior to attempting this exercise, which demands a combination of movement and stabilisation from the abdominals.

It is important that you master your technique prior to introducing an external weight, i.e. dumbbell. Assume a position on the ball where by the upper part of your trunk is slightly arched backwards. Do not go too far to begin with, as this will be an unfamiliar range to control at first.

Your 'anchor' will be provided by your own stabilising muscles, so it is not advisable to fix your feet under a weight, or to have someone hold your feet down for you. Begin with the lower stomach flat, then gently exhale and imagine your ribs pulling towards your pelvis. Keep your chin tucked in as your shoulders rise to just above level with your hips. Keep focusing on stomach flattening as you lower your back down again.

This exercise can also be done on a slight diagonal, by beginning with one elbow pointing down towards the floor, and finishing with that same elbow pointing across the opposite hip.

It must be reinforced that in order to perform these exercises correctly, a great deal of core stability is necessary. They in no way replace other core exercises, but offer a sports specific option to those athletes who require strength in greater range than normal.

These are only a few examples of how the exercise ball can be used for weight training, but by reviewing the principles above, you may find that the ball can enhance your normal programme and improve the way in which your body responds to external loading.

Bibliography

Bartonietz, K. & Strange, D.: 1998. The use of Swiss Balls in athletic training: an effective combination of load and fun. *IAAF Quarterly*, **2**: 35–41.

Borghuis, J., Hof, A.L. & Lemmink, K.A.: 2008. The importance of sensory-motor control in providing core stability: implications for measurement and training. *Sports Med.*, **38**(11): 893–916.

Bullock-Saxton, J., Janda, V. & Bullock, M.: 1993. Reflex activation of gluteal muscles in walking: an approach to restoration of muscle function for patients with low back pain. *Spine*, **18**(6): 704–708.

Carpes, F.P., Reinehr, F.B. & Mota, C.B.: 2008. Effects of a program for trunk strength and stability on pain, low back and pelvis kinematics, and body balance: a pilot study. *J. Body Movt. Ther.*, **12**(1): 22–30.

Carriere, B.: 1993. Swiss Ball exercises. *PT Magazine*, September.

Critchley, D.: 2002. Instructing pelvic floor contraction facilitates transversus abdominis thickness increase during low-abdominal hollowing. *Physiother. Res. Int.*, **27**(2): 65–75.

Dickerman, R.D., Smith, A. & Stevens, Q.E.: 2004. Umbilical and bilateral inguinal hernias in a veteran powerlifter: is it a pressure-overload syndrome? *Clinical Journal of Sport Medicine*, **14**(2): 95–6.

Foxhoven, B. & Plate, P.: 1996. Athletes with back pain: a trunk stabilization program. Strength and Conditioning Journal, 69–73.

Geraci, M.C. Jr. & Brown, W.: 2005. Evidence-based treatment of hip and pelvic injuries in runners. *Phys. Med. Rehabil. Clin. N. Am.* **16**(3): 711–47.

Gracovetsky, S.A .: 1997. Linking the Spinal Engine With the Legs: a Theory of Human Gait, in Vleeming, A., Mooney, V., Dorman, T., Snijders, C. & Stoeckart, R.: 1997. *Movement, Stability and Low Back Pain: the Essential Role of the Pelvis.* Churchill Livingstone, Edinburgh.

Grenier, S.G. & McGill, S.M.: 2007. Quantification of lumbar stability by using two different abdominal activation strategies. *Arch. Phys. Med. Rehabil.* **88**(1): 54–62.

Hides, J.A., Richardson, C.A. & Jull, G.A.: 1996. Multifidus recovery is not automatic following resolution of acute first-episode low back pain. *Spine*, **21**(23): 2763–9.

Hides, J.A., Stanton, W.R., McMahon, S., Sims, K. & Richardson, C.A.: 2008. Effect of stabilization training on multifidus muscle cross-sectional area among young elite cricketers with low back pain. *J. Orthop. Sports Phys. Ther.*, Mar, **38**(3): 101–8.

Hodges, P. & Richardson, C.A.: 1997. Feedforward contraction of transversus abdominis is not influenced by the direction of arm movement. *Experimental Brain Research*, **114**(2): 362–70.

Hodges, P.: 2001. Changes in motor planning of feedforward postural responses of the trunk muscles in low back pain. *Experimental Brain Research*, **141**(2): 261–6.

Hodges, P.W., Heijnen, I. & Gandevia, S.C.: 2001. Postural activity of the diaphragm is reduced in humans when respiratory demand increases. *Journal of Physiology*, **537**(3): 999–1008.

Hodges, P.W., Gurfinkel, V.S., Brumagne, S., Smith, T.C. & Cordo, P.C.: 2002. Coexistence of stability and mobility in postural control: evidence from postural compensation for respiration. *Experimental Brain Research*, **144**(3): 293–302.

Kapandji, I.A.: 1982. *The Physiology of the Joints, Vols. 1–3.* Churchill Livingstone, Edinburgh.

Koumantakis, G.A., Watson, P.J. & Oldham, J.A.: 2005. Trunk muscle stabilization training plus general exercise versus general exercise only: randomized controlled trial of patients with recurrent low back pain. *Phys Ther.*, Mar, **85**(3): 209–25.

Lee, D.: 1997. Instability of the Sacroiliac Joint and the Consequences of Gait, in Vleeming, A., Mooney, V., Dorman, T., Snijders, C. & Stoeckart, R.: 1997. *Movement, Stability and Low Back Pain: the Essential Role of the Pelvis.* Churchill Livingstone, Edinburgh.

Lee, D.G., Lee, L.J. & McLaughlin, L.: 2008. Stability, continence and breathing: the role of fascia following pregnancy and delivery. *J. Body Movt. Ther.,* **12**(4): 333–48.

Leetun, D.T., Ireland, M.L., Willson, J.D., Ballantyne, B.T. & Davis, I.M.: 2004. Core stability measures as risk factors for lower extremity injury in athletes. *Med. Sci. Sports Exerc.,* **36**(6): 926–34.

Lippincott, Williams & Wilkins: 1999. First randomized trial of treatments for groin pain. *Sports Medicine Digest,* **21**(3): 25–30.

Marshall, P.W. & Murphy, B.A.: 2006. Evaluation of functional and neuromuscular changes after exercise rehabilitation for low back pain using a Swiss Ball: a pilot study. *J. Manipulative Physiol. Ther.,* **29**(7): 550–60.

Marshall, P.W. & Murphy, B.A.: 2008. Muscle activation changes after exercise rehabilitation for chronic low back pain. *Arch. Phys. Med. Rehabil.,* **89**(7): 1305–13.

Mottram, S. & Comerford, M.: 1998. Stability, dysfunction and low back pain. *J. of Orthopedic Medicine,* **20**(2):13–18.

Norris, C.M.: 1994. Abdominal training: dangers and exercise modifications. *Physiotherapy in Sport,* **19**(5): 10–13.

O'Sullivan, P.B. & Beales, D.J.: 2007. Changes in pelvic floor and diaphragm kinematics and respiratory patterns in subjects with sacroiliac joint pain following a motor learning intervention: a case series. *Man Ther.,* **12**(3): 209–18.

Reeve, A. & Dilley, A.: 2009. Effects of posture on the thickness of transversus abdominis in pain-free subjects. *Man. Ther.,* May, **12**. [Epub ahead of print]

Richardson, C.A. & Jull, G.A.: 1994. Concepts of Assessment and Rehabilitation for Active Lumbar Stability, in Boyling, J. and Palastanga, N. Grieve's *Modern Manual Therapy.* Churchill Livingstone, Edinburgh.

Richardson, C.A. & Jull, G.A.: 1995. Muscle control – pain control. What exercises would you prescribe? *Manual Therapy,* **1**: 1–9.

Sell, T., Tsai, Y., Smoglia, J., Myers, J. & Lephart S.: 2007. Strength, flexibility and balance characteristics of highly proficient golfers. *J. Strength and Conditioning Research,* **21**(4): 1166–1171.

Teyhen, D.S., Rieger, J.L., Westrick, R.B., Miller, A.C., Molloy, J.M. & Childs, J.D.: 2008. Changes in deep abdominal muscle thickness during common trunk-strengthening exercises using ultrasound imaging. *J. Orthop. Sports Phys. Ther.,* **38**(10): 596–605.

Thompson, C.J., Cobb, K.M. & Blackwell, J.: 2007. Functional training improves club head speed and functional fitness in older golfers. *J. Strength Cond. Res.,* **21**(1):131–7.

Willson, J.D., Dougherty, C.P., Ireland, M.L. & Davis, I.M.: 2005. Core stability and its relationship to lower extremity function and injury. *J. Am. Acad. Orthop. Surg.,* **13**(5):316–25.

Zazulak, B.T., Hewett, T.E., Reeves, N.P., Goldberg, B. & Cholewicki, J.: 2007. Deficits in neuromuscular control of the trunk predict knee injury risk: a prospective biomechanical-epidemiologic study. Am. *J. Sports Med.,* **35**(7):1123–30.

The Anatomy of Stretching
Brad Walker

978 1 905367 03 0 (UK)/978 1 55643 596 (US); **£14.99/$24.95**; 176 pages; 265 mm x 194 mm; 320 colour illustrations; paperback

Books on stretching are common, but *The Anatomy of Stretching* takes a more fundamental approach than the others, taking the reader inside the body to show exactly what is happening during a stretch. At the heart of the book are 300 full-colour illustrations that show the primary and secondary muscles worked in 114 key stretches arranged by body area. Author Brad Walker brings years of expertise – he works with elite-level and world-champion athletes, and lectures on injury prevention – to this how-to guide. He looks at stretching from every angle, including physiology and flexibility; the benefits of stretching; the different types of stretching; rules for safe stretching; and how to stretch properly. Aimed at fitness enthusiasts of any level, as well as at fitness pros, *The Anatomy of Stretching* also focuses on which stretches are useful for the alleviation or rehabilitation of specific sports injuries.

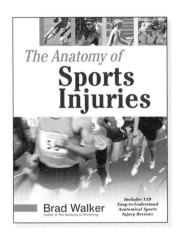

The Anatomy of Sports Injuries
Brad Walker

978 1 905367 06 1 (UK)/ 978 1 55643 666 6 (US); **£16.99/$29.95**; 256 pages; 265 mm x 194 mm; 250 colour / black and white illustrations; paperback

The Anatomy of Sports Injuries takes you inside the body to show exactly what is happening when a sports injury occurs. At the heart of *The Anatomy of Sports Injuries* are 300 full-colour illustrations that show the sports injury in detail, along with 200 line drawings of simple stretching, strengthening, and rehabilitation exercises that the reader can use to speed up the recovery process. *The Anatomy of Sports Injuries* is for every sports player or fitness enthusiast who has been injured and would like to know what the injury involves, how to rehabilitate the area, and how to prevent complications or injury in the future. This book is the perfect partner for Brad's other book, *The Anatomy of Stretching*.

Brad Walker, B.Sc. Health Sciences, is a prominent Australian sports trainer with more than 20 years experience in the health and fitness industry. He graduated from the University of New England, and has postgraduate accreditations in athletics, swimming, and triathlon coaching.

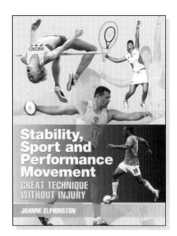

Stability, Sport, and Performance Movement

Joanne Elphinston

978 1 905367 09 2 (UK)/978 1 55643 746 5 (US); **£24.99/$32.95**; 352 pages; 265 mm x 194 mm; 320 colour illustrations; paperback

In every sport, there are athletes who represent true technical excellence. Their movement seems effortless, controlled and efficient: they create and control forces in the most effective way.

The building blocks of stability, mobility, symmetry, and balance provide the foundation for sports movement development and injury resistance. These elements combine to prevent the physical restrictions, imbalances and inefficient muscle recruitment patterns which can block athletes from meeting their movement goals. The right muscles firing at the right time and in the right sequence can enable athletes to achieve their full physical potential.

Full of colour photographs and images to illustrate the techniques and theories involved, *Stability, Sport, and Performance Movement* introduces functional stability principles as they apply to sporting movement. A comprehensive chapter on movement testing is followed with four chapters of integrated exercise techniques, which clearly demonstrate form and progression from early activation through to high-level neuromuscular drills. Programmes and clinical examples help the reader to appreciate the application of this approach across a variety of sports.

It is an approach that has been used with international-level athletes in disciplines as diverse as swimming, badminton, gymnastics, karate, cycling, weight lifting, basketball, athletics, snow sports, football, golf, equestrian sports, and tennis. However, it is applicable and relevant across all age groups and ability levels, from beginners through to veterans. Effective adult movement starts with great foundations, so a dedicated chapter on establishing stable controlled movement in children is included.

Joanne Elphinston, is a Performance Consultant, international lecturer and physiotherapist working with elite and professional athletes including Olympic, Commonwealth and World Championship medallists, Premiership footballers and professional golfers. Joanne is a consultant on Performance Movement to the British Olympic Association, as well as advising professional sporting organisations on technical movement enhancement for performance, injury prevention and rehabilitation. She also has extensive experience in child and adolescent movement development for sport and its progression into senior competition.